Dirty KETO

How to Cheat Without Getting Caught

NEW YORK TIMES BESTSELLING AUTHOR

E.K. BLAIR

and ERIKA RIVERA

Dirty KETO

DEDIC

To my husband, son, and daughter

Without your support, this dream come true would still be just a dream.

Erika

ATION

To Sally and Kylie

This is all your fault.

E. K.

CONT

ENTS

INTROD

The thought of embarking on a weight-loss journey is scary. There are so many changes that one must make in order to lower that number on the scale. It can seem overwhelming, impossible even. I mean, how is a person supposed to live without tater tots or chocolate cake? Are we really supposed to ignore our cravings and never give in? And what about the guilt? How do you get back on track after diving face-first into a plate of biscuits and gravy?

If only there were a way to cheat and not get caught by that pesky bathroom scale.

Let's get real, nobody wants to see that number creep up. No one wants to suck in and hold their breath while trying to squeeze into a pair of pants.

So, what if I told you that you could still enjoy some yummy *junk* food while losing weight?

Would you believe me?

You should! Let me tell you why.

95 pounds ago, I was miserable and told myself I would do anything to lose the weight, as long as I did not have to give up my favorite foods. You know the ones I'm talking about: breads, pastas, cookies, and cocktails. Okay, maybe not the cocktails, because I don't like the taste of alcohol, but my good friend, Erika, does. After a long day at the office and taking care of her two teenagers, the girl needs a drink! She may need a chunk of her yummy no-bake peanut butter bars as well. Let's face it, life is stressful, and food serves as a comfort. Some say it's more satisfying than sex, and when you taste Erika's no-bake peanut butter bar recipe, I think you might just agree. I should also mention that Erika was able to indulge on those treats while losing 40 pounds!

Between the two of us, we have dropped 135 pounds.

Let me be clear, we didn't do it by eating the recipes in this book on a daily occurrence.

I wish!

Nope, that isn't what this cookbook is.

This is the cookbook you are going to open up when you're needing a good cheat meal. You know the kind I'm talking about.

Dirty.

Filthy.

UCTION

Sexy.

Okay, so maybe you wouldn't classify a chili cheese dog as sexy, but it sure is dirty and that's exactly how Erika and I like our food.

But to successfully lose weight, you will have to eat clean the majority of the time and track those macros! Go to any bookstore and you'll find shelves filled with clean keto cookbooks. They'll discuss the benefits of grass-fed beef and free-range eggs. They'll talk about fasting and autophagy. They'll toss around terms like, certified organic, vegetarian-fed, and omega-3 enriched.

Zzzz . . .

Sorry, that was so boring that I dozed off for a second.

You won't find any of that in this book, I promise.

Now, let me just state for the record that neither Erika and myself are nutritionists or doctors, we are not experts in this field, and we're definitely not refined chefs.

We are just two girls who ventured on a weight-loss journey and found our own path to success.

You want to know how we did it?

Okay, here is our secret. Our dirty little secret.

We are cheaters.

There, I said it.

We cheat.

Not all the time; only when we are on the verge of falling off the weight-loss wagon.

This book is filled with some of our favorite cheat recipes while keeping it low carb and keto—*dirty* keto! (I will explain more about what that means a little later.)

Let me first rewind and introduce the two of us. Don't worry, I'll keep this part short and sweet.

My name is E.K. Blair, and I am hanging on to the age of 39 as if my life depended on it. I am a wife to an amazing man, and together we have an 11-year old son and an 8-year daughter. I am also a New York Times bestselling author. I write young adult, new adult contemporary romance, and suspense novels. My life is chaotic and busy here in Oklahoma, but I am happy and healthy, so I can't complain.

Now, let me introduce Erika. She asked me to write this for her because, well, writing is sort of my thing. I met Erika a couple years ago through Instagram. I know, we are total millennials. Don't judge!

Erika is a 37-year-old California girl, wife, and mother. She has a 15-year-old daughter and a 13-year-old son and trust me when I say that they keep her on her toes. Her days are spent working as a clinical medical assistant, and she is also a certified phlebotomist.

What's a certified phlebotomist, you ask?

I have no clue, so hold on while I Google that . . .

Okay, I'm back. So, basically, she deals with blood, and that's all I'm going to say because, *eww*. Let's get back to food, shall we?

So, Erika and I connected through keto. We were posting photos of the meals we were eating and messaging each other for the recipes. After a while, we decided to gather up our recipes, write a book, and share them all with you! We wanted to show our true authentic selves and not hide behind the false image of perfection. No, we don't eat clean and perfect all the time. Yes, we have days that don't go the way we would have hoped. We struggle with body image and that damn number on the scale. And, yes, there are times when we really miss the filthy foods of our past. The cobblers, the bagels, and the martinis. *I'm speaking for Erika on that last one!*

What I'm trying to say is, we are real, we are messy, and we want to show you how you can cheat and not get caught!

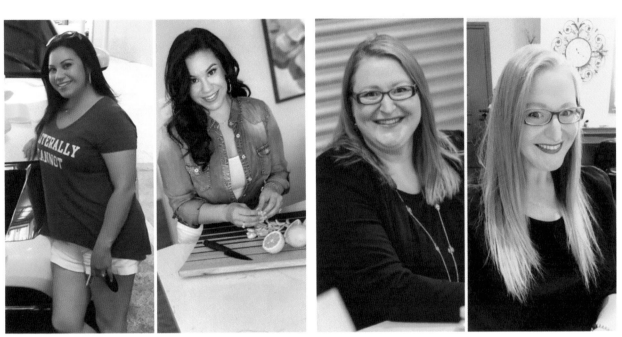

Erika   E.K.

You've probably heard about clean keto, lazy keto, and dirty keto, but what exactly do they mean? Look, I'm no expert, but I'm going to break it down for you as simple as possible. No need for any scientific research references here.

Let's jump right in!

What is ketosis?

This is when the body stops using carbohydrates for energy and starts using fat. To achieve ketosis, the formula is quite simple:

5% of your diet comes from carbs

20% of your diet comes from protein

75% of your diet comes from fat

And if you are wanting to lose weight, just make sure you are in a calorie deficit.

So, when you hear the term macros, this is what it means. Your macros are carbohydrates, protein, and fat.

What is the keto diet?

The ketogenic diet is a very low carb, high fat diet that puts your body into a state of ketosis. It is a great option for those looking to lose weight and/or manage Type 2 Diabetes. In my case (E.K.), I was able to reverse my Type 2 Diabetes and lower my cholesterol. There are so many benefits to this particular way of eating, but it can feel overwhelming at first. It's also important to note that one size doesn't fit all, and you will need to adapt the diet to fit your lifestyle in a way in which you are still seeing results. There is a big misconception that the ketogenic diet will severely limit the types of foods you can eat. This is simply not true. In fact, I have found keto to be extremely flexible, but it all depends on how you keto.

Clean Keto

This is exactly what it sounds like, clean eating. The focus with clean keto is to consume nutrient-dense whole foods of high quality. What do I mean by *high quality*? I'm talking about grass-fed beef, wild-caught seafood, free-range eggs. Clean keto also restricts the consumption of processed foods, although can still be eaten in moderation. With this way of eating, it is important to track the macros you are consuming.

Lazy Keto

If you do not like tracking macros or weighing and measuring your food, then you should try lazy keto. Your goal is to eat no more than 20 grams of carbohydrates in a given day without counting calories or tracking macros.

T DIRTY

Dirty Keto

This is exactly what it sounds like. Dirty keto strays from the clean eating described above. The quality of food is lower and includes heavily processed items such as pre-packaged snacks and fast food. You should track your calories and macros when eating dirty keto because it is easy to gain weight if you are not careful.

Why Erika and I chose to be dirty?

Because we can't live without yummy, delicious processed foods.

Seriously though, the two of us had the same goal, lose weight, and keep it off.

In order to achieve the latter, we knew we had to modify the keto diet in a way that it would fit our hectic lifestyles and also be sustainable. Let's get real, if you told me that I could only eat clean keto, I would've crashed and burned two week in! I don't know about you, but I have a major junk food tooth, and when I get cravings, they are so hard to ignore. Plus, if this was how I planned on eating for the long term, I didn't want to feel deprived.

So, dirty keto it was!

Now, do Erika and I eat dirty for every meal? No.

Do we eat it every day? Aside from the Skinny Syrups we use in our coffee, no.

Do we eat dirty every week? Heck yeah, we do!

In the end, it really doesn't matter how you keto just as long as you are reaching your goals and seeing results. They key is to find a lifestyle that makes you happy and that is easily sustainable. So, make whatever tweaks you feel are necessary, but also remember that to see changes, you have to make changes, and some of those changes are going to be uncomfortable. Just don't make yourself too uncomfortable to the point that you give up. Oh, and don't listen to any negativity around you. Everyone's weight-loss journey is going to look different, and that is okay! It is all about what works best for you!

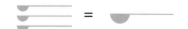

3 teaspoons   1 tablespoon

2 tablespoons   1/8 cup   1 fluid oz.

4 tablespoons   1/4 cup

5 tablespoons + 1 teaspoon   1/3 cup

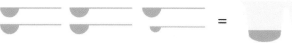

8 tablespoons   1/2 cup

10 tablespoons + 2 teaspoon   2/3 cup

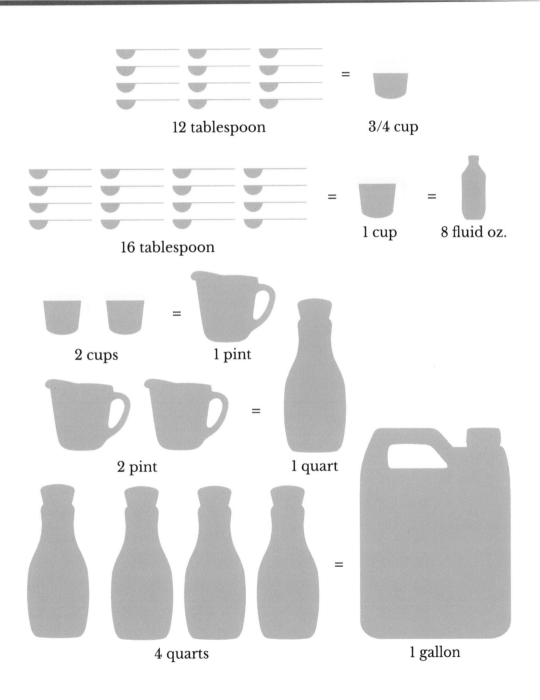

12 tablespoon = 3/4 cup

16 tablespoon = 1 cup = 8 fluid oz.

2 cups = 1 pint

2 pint = 1 quart

4 quarts = 1 gallon

DIRTY FA

Baking Flours

Almond Flour

Almond Meal

Coconut Flour

Psyllium Husk Powder

Walnut Flour

Baking Mixes

CarbQuik

Good Dee's

Highkey

Keto and Co.

Kiss My Keto

Lakanto

Pyure

Swerve Sweets

Breads & Buns

Chompies

Great Low Carb Bread Company

Kiss My Keto

Rays the Valley

Smart Baking Company

Sola Bread Co.

ThinSlim Foods

Chocolate

Bake Believe

ChocZero

Hershey's Sugar Free

Kiss My Keto

Lakanto

Lily's Sweets

Russell Stover Sugar Free

Simply Lite Chocolate

Milk Alternatives

Almond Milk

Cashew Milk

Coconut Milk

Fairlife Lactose-Free Milk

Half & Half

Heavy Whipping Cream

Macadamia Milk

Soy Milk

Oils & Fats

Avocado Oil

Bacon Fat

Butter

Coconut Oil

Duck Fat

Extra Virgin Olive Oil

Ghee

Macadamia Oil

MCT Oil

Palm Oil

Sesame Oil

Tallow

Pizza & Pastas

Better Than Foods

Cali'flour Foods

Great Low Carb Bread Company

Healthy Noodles

Kbosh Artisan Keto

Liviva

Outer Aisle Pizza Crusts

Rays the Valley

ThinSlim Foods Im*pasta*bles

VORITES

Sugar Alternatives

Lakanto Classic Granular Monk Fruit Sweetener

Lakanto Golden Monk Fruit Sweetener

Lakanto Powdered Monk Fruit Sweetener

Lakanto Liquid Monk Fruit Extract

Madhava Organic Agave Five

Pyure Stevia Blend

Pyure Liquid Stevia Extract

Pyure Harmless Honey

Stevia

Sukrin Monk Fruit

Sukrin Gold

Swerve Brown Sugar Replacement

Swerve Granular Sugar Replacement

Swerve Confectioner's Sugar Replacement

Truvia Sugar Blend

Truvia Brown Sugar Blend

Truvia Confectioners

Truvia Sweet Complete

Truvia Organic Liquid Sweetener

Wholesome Allulose Liquid Sweetener

Wholesome Allulose Granular Sweetener

Syrups & Flavor Extracts

ChocZero

Jordan's Skinny Mixes

Maple Grove Farms Sugar Free Maple Syrup

McCormick Extracts & Flavors

Mrs. Butterworth's Sugar Free Pancake Syrup

One on One Flavors

Smucker's Sugar Free Pancake Syrup

Torani Sugar Free Syrups

Walden Farms

Tortillas & Wraps

Cut Da Carb Flatbread

Joseph's Lavash Wraps

La Banderita Carb Counter Tortillas

La Tortilla Low Carb Tortillas

Mama Lupe's Low Carb Tortillas

Mission Carb Balance Tortillas

Mr. Tortilla

Ole Xtreme

WALK OF

Biscuits & Gravy

Pizza Baked Eggs

Breakfast Casserole

Pancake Stack with Blueberry Compote

Waffle-wich

Stuffed French Toast

SHAME

Blueberry Bagels

Everything Bagels

Gingerbread Bagels

Banana Chocolate Chip Waffles

Bacon, Egg, and Cheese
McMorning After

Monkey Bread

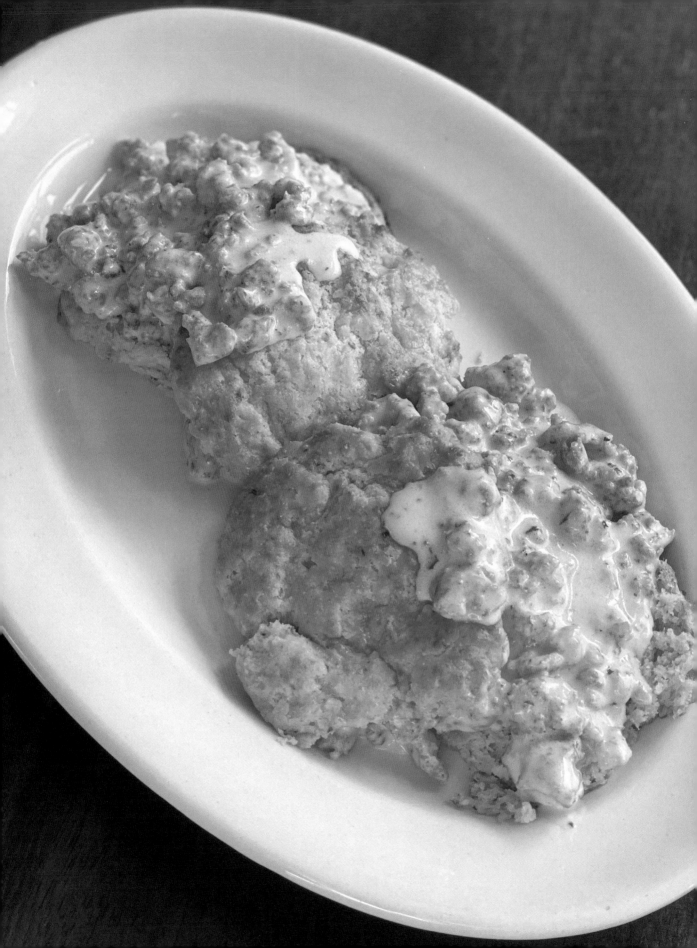

Prep Time: 15 minutes
Cook Time: 10 minutes
Yield: 10 servings

BISCUITS & GRAVY

Ingredients

BISCUITS

2 cups almond flour
3 eggs
½ cup sour cream
1 tablespoon baking powder
1 tablespoon granular sweetener
1 teaspoon salt
8 tablespoons of cold butter, cubed

GRAVY

1 pound ground sausage
2 ounces cream cheese
½ cup heavy cream
1 teaspoon salt
½ teaspoon pepper
1 teaspoon onion powder
1 teaspoon garlic powder
Parsley for garnish

Directions

1. Preheat oven to 400°F and line a baking sheet with parchment paper.
2. In a medium mixing bowl, add all ingredients for the biscuits, except the butter. Stir together, careful not to overmix.
3. Add cold butter and gently combine.
4. Drop the dough, in even portions, onto the baking sheet to make 10 biscuits and bake for 8-10 minutes.
5. For the gravy, brown the sausage in a large skillet and drain excess grease.
6. Add the cream cheese and melt before whisking in the heavy whipping cream, salt, pepper, onion powder, and garlic powder.
7. Spoon gravy over warm biscuits and enjoy.

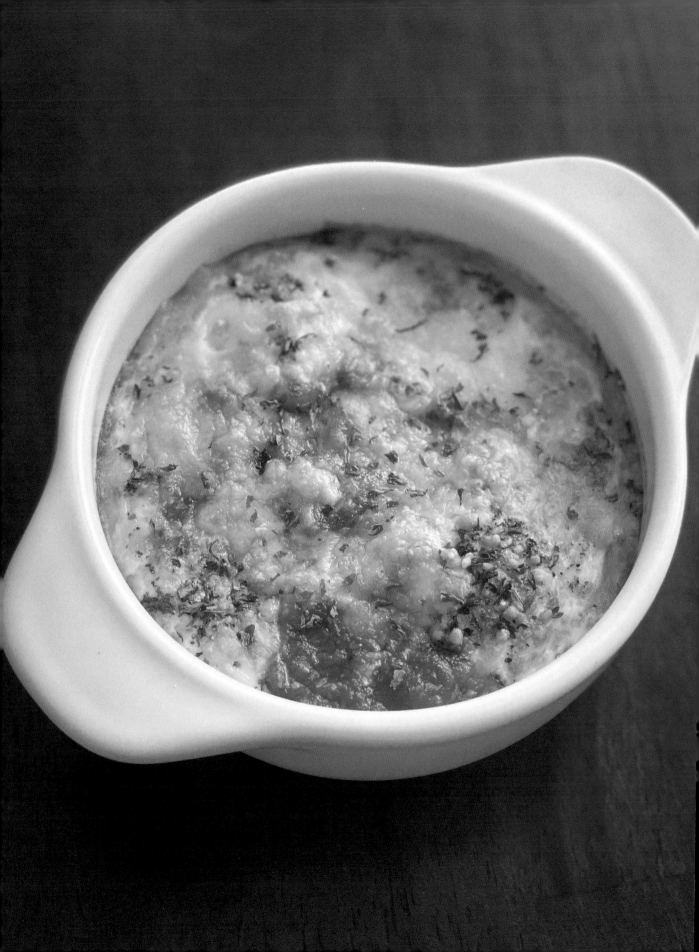

Prep Time: 5 minutes
Cook Time: 15 minutes
Yield: 1 serving

PIZZA BAKED EGGS

Ingredients

2 eggs
¼ cup Rao's no-sugar-added marinara sauce
2 tablespoons parmesan cheese
2 tablespoons mozzarella cheese
Salt and pepper to taste
1 tablespoon fresh or dried parsley for garnish

Directions

1. Preheat oven to 375°F and grease a single-serving baking dish.
2. Spread 2 tablespoons of marinara sauce on the bottom of the baking dish.
3. Sprinkle 1 tablespoon of parmesan cheese and 1 tablespoon of mozzarella cheese on top of the sauce.
4. Crack the eggs on top of cheese and season with salt and pepper.
5. Spread remaining sauce over the eggs.
6. Top with remaining parmesan and mozzarella cheese and garnish with parsley.
7. Bake for 12-15 minutes.

Pro Tip

Add in your favorite pizza toppings.

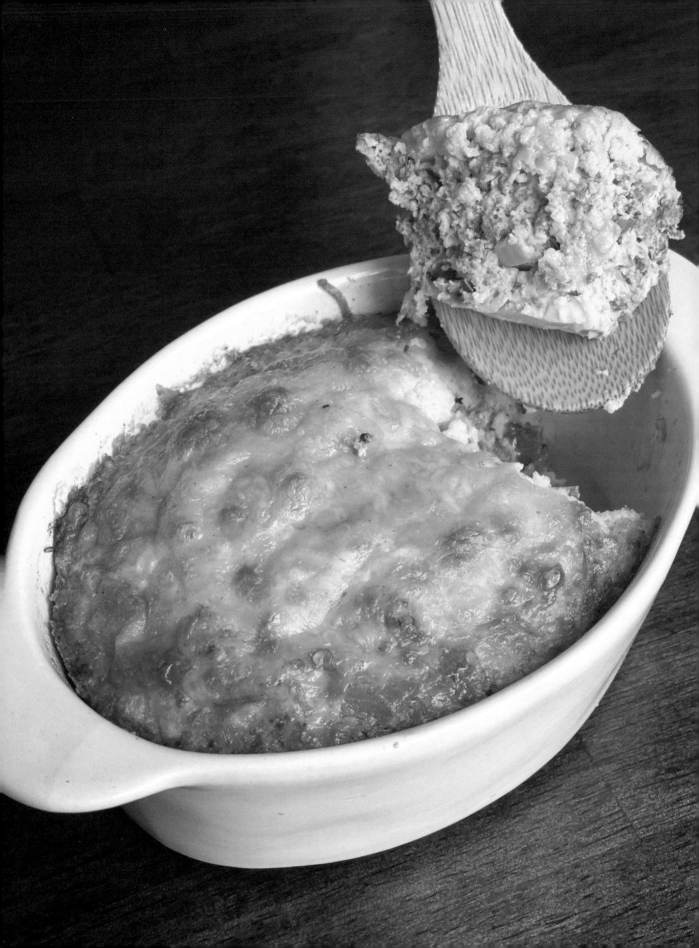

BREAKFAST CASSEROLE

Ingredients

24 ounces pork sausage

1 medium red bell pepper, chopped

½ medium white onion, chopped

1 bag frozen riced cauliflower, cooked and drained

2 cups shredded cheddar cheese

1 ¼ cups Carbquik baking mix

2 cups unsweetened almond milk

4 eggs at room temperature

¼ teaspoon pepper

Directions

1. Preheat oven to 400°F and grease a 9x12 baking dish.
2. Using a large skillet, cook sausage, bell pepper, and onion until sausage is no longer pink. Drain grease.
3. In a 9x12 baking dish, combine the sausage mixture, riced cauliflower, and 2 cups of cheese.
4. Whisk together the Carbquik, eggs, almond milk, and pepper in a mixing bowl and then pour into the baking dish.
5. Cover and refrigerate overnight.
6. Bake, uncovered, at 400°F for 40 minutes. Top with remaining cheese and continue to bake for 10-15 minutes.

Pro Tip

In a bowl, pour warm water over eggs for 15 minutes to bring to room temperature.

WALK OF SHAME

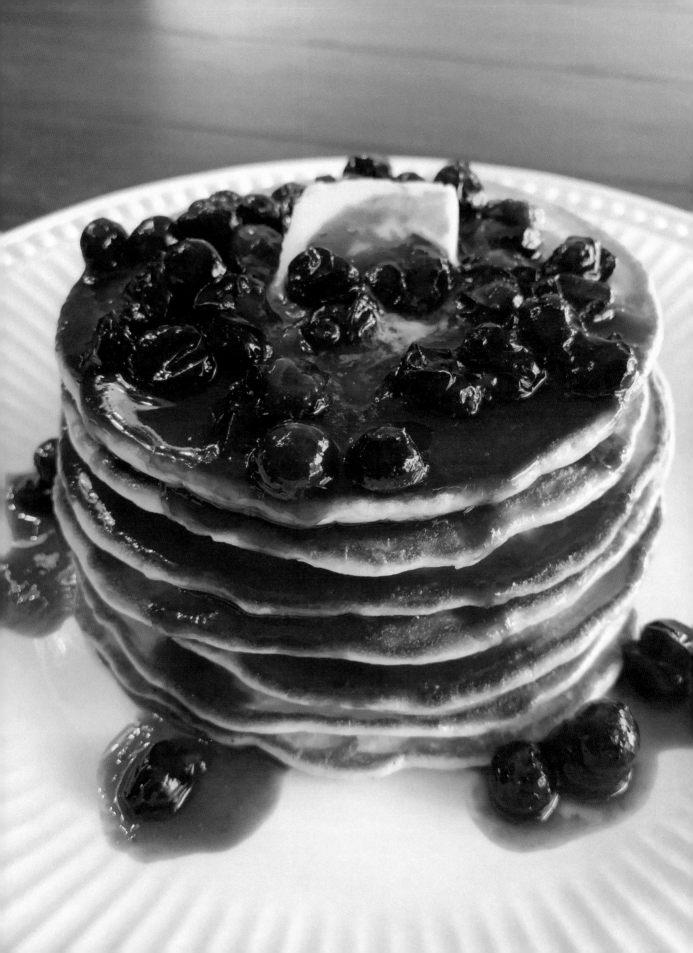

PANCAKE STACK WITH BLUEBERRY COMPOTE

Ingredients

PANCAKES

4 eggs, room temperature
4 ounces cream cheese, softened
¾ cup almond flour
1 teaspoon vanilla
1 teaspoon baking powder
1-2 tablespoons granular sweetener
1-2 tablespoons butter

BLUEBERRY COMPOTE

1 cup blueberries
1 teaspoon granular sweetener

Directions

1. In a blender, mix all ingredients for 1-2 minutes. Let sit for 10 minutes.
2. Using a skillet or griddle on medium heat, melt butter. When hot, pour ¼ cup of batter onto surface and cook for about 2 minutes until bubbles form in the batter. Flip and cook for another 2 minutes.
3. For the compote, mix blueberries and sweetener in a small, microwave-safe bowl. Microwave in 15-second intervals until berries burst. This will take less than a minute.
4. Pour over pancakes.

Pro Tip

Make batter ahead of time and store in the fridge for a quick and easy breakfast.

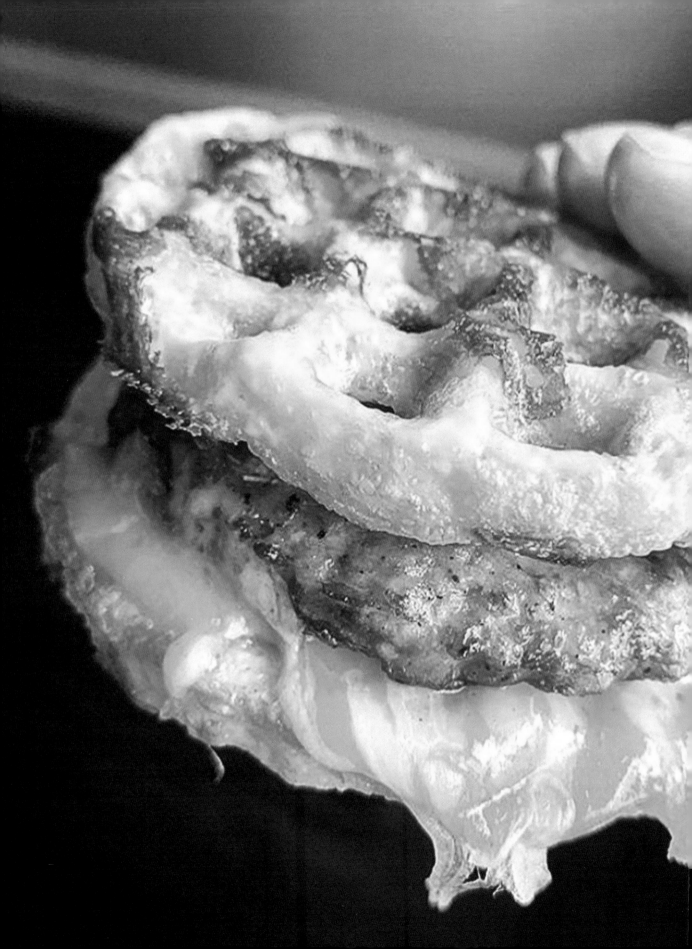

Prep Time: 3 minutes
Cook Time: 10 minutes
Yield: 1 serving

WAFFLE-WICH

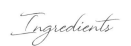

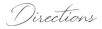

2 eggs
1 teaspoon almond flour
2 teaspoons cheddar cheese, shredded
1 sausage patty
1 slice American cheese

1. Heat a mini waffle iron on medium-high heat.
2. Crack 1 egg and lightly beat with a fork. Stir in almond flour.
3. When waffle iron is ready, sprinkle approximately ½ teaspoon of shredded cheese directly onto the waffle iron and allow to cook for 30 seconds.
4. Pour ½ of the egg batter on top of melted cheese and then top with another ½ teaspoon cheddar cheese. Close the waffle iron and cook until lightly crispy and cook until light turns off
5. Repeat steps 3 and 4 for second waffle.
6. Heat sausage patty and fry 1 egg.
7. Assemble sandwich with sausage, slice of American cheese, and fried egg.

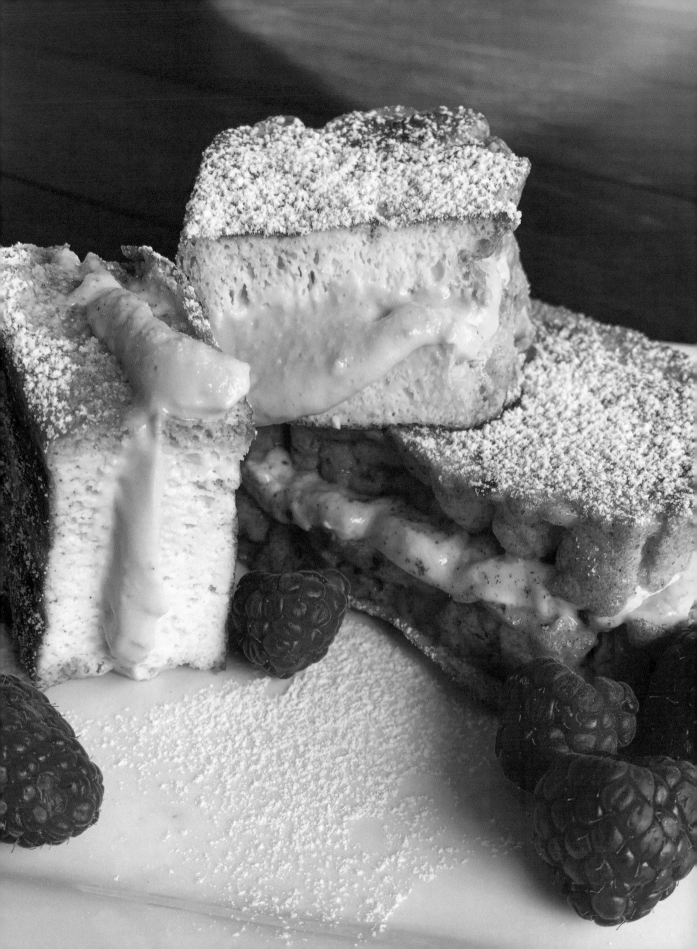

Prep Time: 30 minutes
Cook Time: 10 minutes
Yield: 3 servings

STUFFED FRENCH TOAST

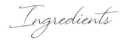 Ingredients

6 slices low-carb bread
3 large eggs
⅓ cup half & half
1 teaspoon vanilla extract
¼ teaspoon ground cinnamon
Pinch of salt

RASPBERRY CREAM CHEESE

½ cup raspberries
2 teaspoons granular sweetener
4 ounces cream cheese, softened
4 tablespoons butter, room temperature
½ teaspoon vanilla extract
1 cup powdered sweetener

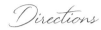 Directions

1. Whisk together eggs, half & half, vanilla extract, ground cinnamon, and salt.
2. Grease griddle or skillet over medium-high heat.
3. Dunk each slice of bread into egg mixture, coating each side. Place in pan and cook until golden on both sides.
4. For the frosting, combine raspberries, granular sweetener, and a splash of water in a small saucepan on medium-low heat. Stir every few minutes, careful to not burn, until the mixture reduces and thickens. This should take around 20 minutes. Remove from heat and allow to cool.
5. In a large mixing bowl, beat together with an electric hand mixer the butter and cream cheese until smooth. Add the raspberry mixture and vanilla, beating until combined.
6. Gradually add in the powdered sweetener until creamy.
7. Stuff the frosting between two slices of French toast and enjoy!

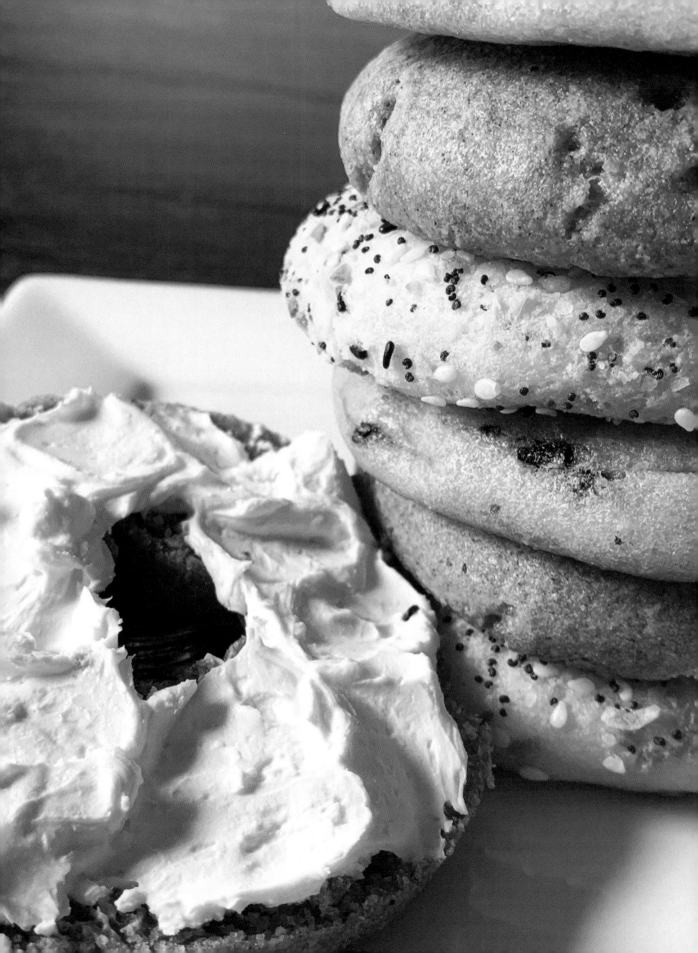

Prep Time: 20 minutes
Cook Time: 17 minutes
Yield: 6 servings

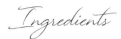

MÉNAGE À TROIS BAGELS

BLUEBERRY BAGELS

2 cups shredded mozzarella cheese
2 ounces cream cheese
1 egg
2 teaspoons baking powder
1 ½ cups almond flour
1 teaspoon vanilla extract
2 tablespoons granular sweetener
½ cup fresh blueberries

EVERYTHING BAGELS

2 cups shredded mozzarella cheese
2 ounces cream cheese
1 egg
2 teaspoons baking powder
1 cup almond flour
Pinch of salt
Everything But The Bagel seasoning to
    sprinkle over the top of the bagel dough

GINGERBREAD BAGELS

2 cups shredded mozzarella cheese
2 ounces cream cheese
1 egg
2 teaspoons baking powder
1 ¼ cup almond flour
¼ cup packed Swerve brown sugar
    replacement
½ tablespoon ground ginger
½ tablespoon ground nutmeg
½ tablespoon ground cinnamon
¼ tablespoon allspice
pinch of salt

Directions

1. Preheat oven to 350°F and line a baking sheet with parchment paper.
2. In a microwave-safe bowl, melt mozzarella and cream cheese in 30-second intervals, stirring in between until melted. This will take around 1 minute.
3. Add remaining ingredients. Mix with a fork or knead with your hands until thoroughly combined. If dough is super sticky, add a little more almond flour.
4. Chill dough in the fridge for at least 1 hour.
5. Divide dough into 6 parts and form into bagel rings. Place onto baking sheet and bake for 15-18 minutes until lightly golden.

Pro Tip

Store leftover bagels in the freezer as they tend to deflate when stored in the fridge.

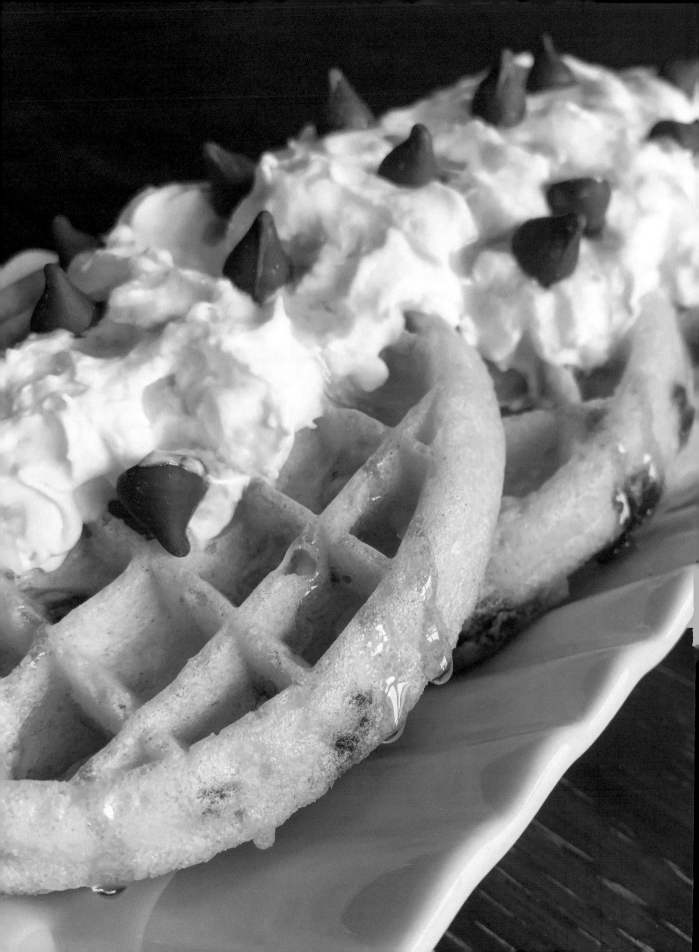

BANANA CHOCOLATE CHIP WAFFLES

Ingredients

1 ¼ cups Carbquik baking mix
1 tablespoon granular sweetener
1 egg, beaten
¼ cup heavy whipping cream
¼ cup unsweetened almond milk
½ teaspoon vanilla extract
½ teaspoon McCormick banana extract
2 tablespoons oil
⅓ cup no-sugar-added chocolate chips

Directions

1. Preheat waffle iron.
2. In a medium mixing bowl, combine together Carbquik and granular sweetener.
3. In a separate bowl, beat egg and heavy cream together using a hand mixer. Stir in almond milk.
4. Pour the wet mixture into your dry ingredient bowl. Add in vanilla and banana extract and oil. Do not overmix. Gently fold in chocolate chips.
5. Pour batter into waffle iron and cook.

WALK OF SHAME

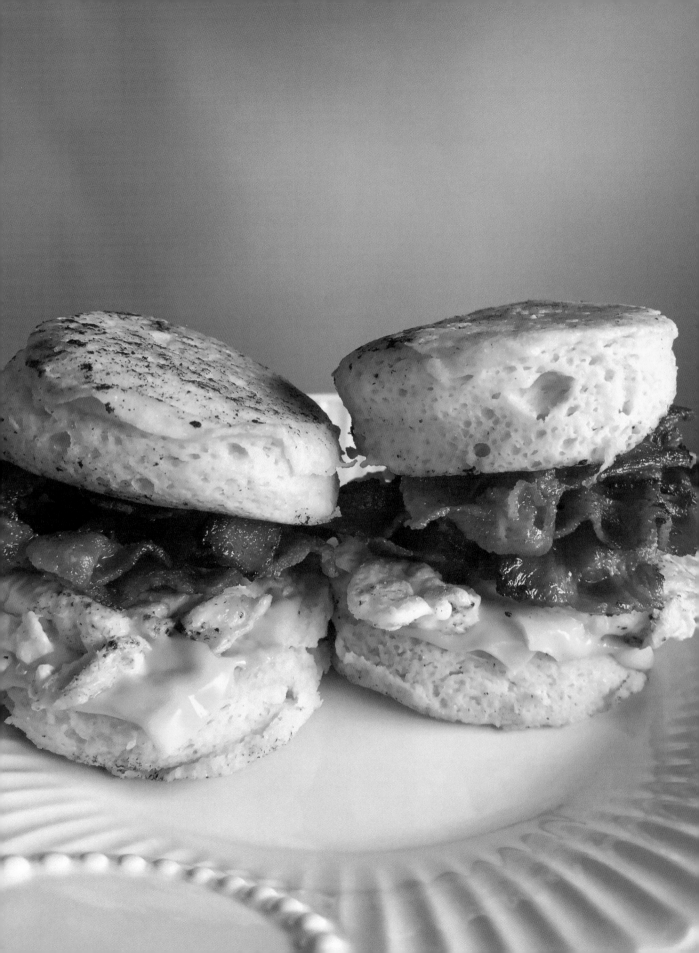

Prep Time: 3 minutes
Cook Time: 5 minutes
Yield: 1 serving

BACON, EGG, AND CHEESE MCMORNING AFTER

Ingredients

1 tablespoon butter, melted
2 eggs (reserve 1 for frying)
½ teaspoon baking powder
3 ½ tablespoons almond flour
1 tablespoon sugar-free pancake syrup
2 slices bacon, pan fried
Cheese

Directions

1. In a mug, mix together melted butter, egg, baking powder, almond flour, and syrup.
2. Place mug in microwave and cook for 90 seconds.
3. Let cool. Slice into two pieces and top with bacon, fried egg, and some cheese.

WALK OF SHAME

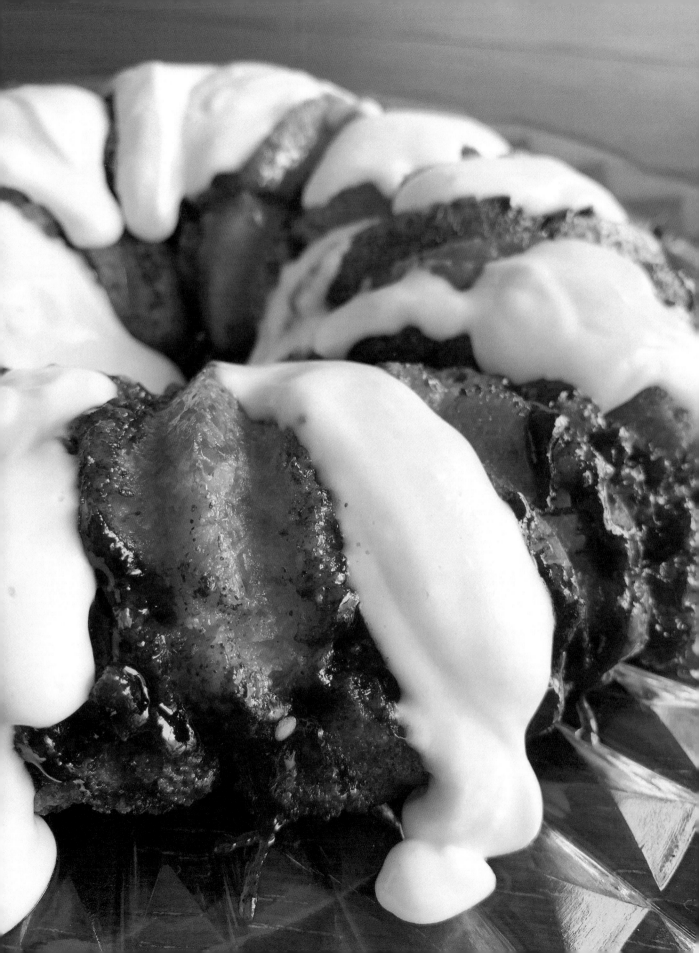

Prep Time: 25 minutes
Cook Time: 35 minutes
Yield: 12 servings

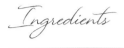

Ingredients

DOUGH

2 cups shredded mozzarella cheese
2 ounces cream cheese
1 egg
1 cup almond flour
1 teaspoon vanilla extract
2 tablespoons granular sweetener

CINNAMON "SUGAR" DUSTING

1 cup granular sweetener
2 teaspoons ground cinnamon

MONKEY SAUCE

½ cup butter
1 cup Swerve brown sugar replacement

CREAM CHEESE ICING

4 ounces cream cheese, softened
4 tablespoons butter, softened
1 cup powdered sweetener
1 teaspoon vanilla extract

Pro Tip

Add in walnuts or pecans for a little crunch!

MONKEY BREAD

Directions

1. Preheat oven to 350°F and grease a Bundt cake pan.
2. In a microwave-safe bowl, melt mozzarella and cream cheese in 30-second intervals, stirring in between until melted. This will take around 1 minute.
3. Add egg, almond flour, vanilla, and granular sweetener. Mix with a fork or knead with your hands until thoroughly combined. If dough is super sticky, add a little more almond flour.
4. Form into a ball, wrap in plastic wrap, and chill dough in the refrigerator until ready to use.
5. For the "sugar" dusting, combine granular sweetener and cinnamon in a large Ziplock bag.
6. Pinch dough off into bite-sized pieces and drop into bag a few at a time. Shake until pieces are coated in the "sugar" mixture. Layer dough balls in a greased Bundt cake pan.
7. In a small saucepan, bring butter and brown sugar replacement to a boil for the monkey sauce. Reduce heat and simmer for 1 to 2 minutes, stirring to avoid burning.
8. Remove from heat and pour over the dough balls.
9. Bake for 35 minutes.
10. In a medium mixing bowl, beat the cream cheese and butter with an electric hand mixer until creamy. Add in the powdered sweetener and vanilla. Continue to beat until smooth,
11. Remove monkey bread from oven and allow to sit for 5 minutes before flipping Bundt pan upside down onto a serving dish and top with frosting.

T E A S

Fathead Dough

Stuffed Mushrooms

Zucchini Bread

Spinach, Artichoke, and Jalapeño Dip

Queso Blanco

Jalapeño Poppers

Maple Mustard Wings

Sticky Peanut Butter & Jelly Wings

Garlicy Lemon Pepper Wings

Elote in a Bowl

Cornbread

Ride 'm Cowboy Pickles

Jalapeño Pimento Cheese

E M E

Oven-Baked Cheese

Party Meatballs

Faux-tato Tots

Jumbo Soft Pretzels

Fried Mozzarella Sticks

Zucchini Fritters

Jicama Fries

Onion Rings

Party Pecans

Chocolate Dipped Bacon

Pecan Praline Bacon

Bourbon Candied Bacon

Fried Pimento Cheese Balls

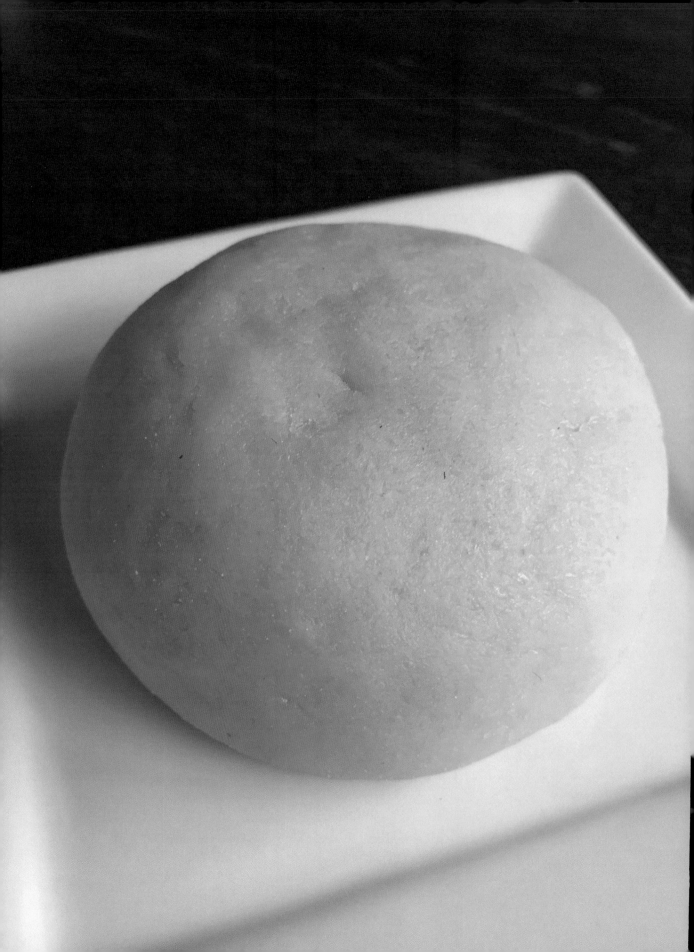

Prep Time: 10 minutes
Cook Time: 0 minutes
Yield: 6 servings

FATHEAD DOUGH

Ingredients

2 cups mozzarella cheese, shredded
2 ounces cream cheese
1 cup almond flour
1 egg

Directions

1. In a microwave safe bowl, melt together the mozzarella cheese and cream cheese by heating in 30-second intervals, stirring in between (approx. 1 minute).
2. With a fork, mix in the almond flour and egg.
3. To full incorporate the ingredients, use your hands to knead dough.
4. Form into a ball, cover in plastic wrap, and chill for at least an hour in the refrigerator.

Pro Tip

You will find many recipes in this book that will call for a prepared batch of fathead dough. This is an extremely versatile dough, so don't be afraid to get creative! Use for bread sticks, dumplings, pie crusts, etc . . .

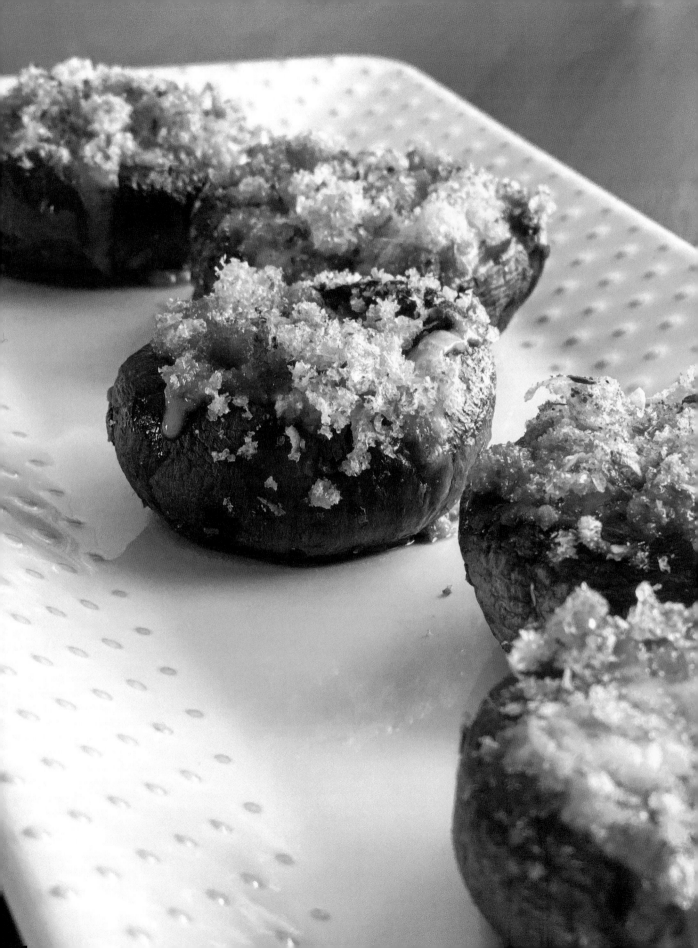

Prep Time: 20 minutes
Cook Time: 15 minutes
Yield: 6 servings

STUFFED MUSHROOMS

Ingredients

2 pounds large mushrooms
1 pound Italian sausage
4 ounces cream cheese, softened
1 tablespoon Italian seasoning
1 teaspoon minced garlic
1 teaspoon salt
½ teaspoon pepper
1 scallion sprig for garnish

TOPPING

3 tablespoons parmesan cheese
¼ cup crushed pork rinds
1 teaspoon Italian seasoning

Directions

1. Preheat oven to 400°F and line a baking sheet with parchment paper.
2. In a skillet, brown the sausage on medium heat. When no pink is left, drain and return to the pan.
3. Add the garlic and cook for 1 minute. Next, add the cream cheese and seasonings. Cook until cheese is melted and ingredients are well combined. Remove from heat and set aside.
4. Clean the mushrooms by wiping the caps of the mushrooms with a damp paper towel. Remove the stems and the brown gills on the inside of the cap.
5. Place mushrooms cap side down on the baking sheet.
6. In a small bowl, stir together the pork rind crumbs, parmesan cheese, and Italian seasoning.
7. Spoon sausage mixture into the mushroom caps and then top with the cheese and pork rind mixture.
8. Bake for 15 minutes until the tops are golden brown.
9. Garnish with scallions and serve.

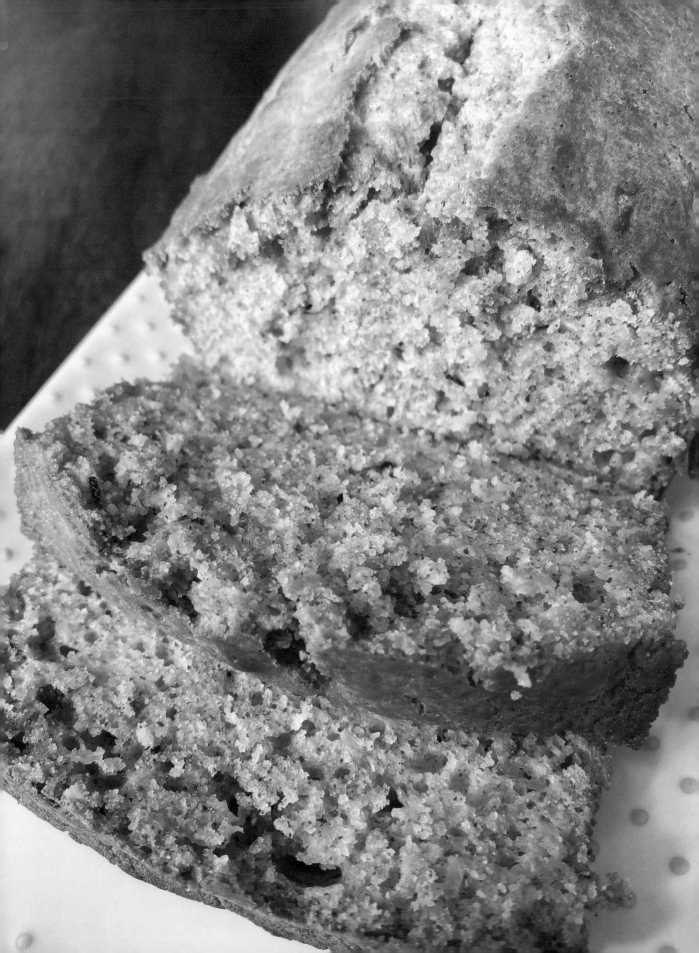

ZUCCHINI BREAD

Ingredients

2 cups almond flour

½ teaspoon salt

½ teaspoon ground cinnamon

½ cup powdered sweetener

1 teaspoon baking soda

2 eggs

4 tablespoons butter, melted

2 medium zucchinis, grated with skin
(approx. 1 ½ cups)

Directions

1. Preheat oven to 350°F and grease a 5x9 bread loaf pan.
2. Using a cheesecloth or dish towel, wrap the grated zucchini and squeeze out as much excess water as you can and set aside.
3. In a large mixing bowl, whisk together the almond flour, salt, cinnamon, powdered sweetener, and baking soda.
4. Add zucchini to the dry ingredients along with the eggs and melted butter. Stir until the batter is well combined.
5. Pour batter into loaf pan and bake for 1 hour or until a toothpick comes out clean. Allow to cool before slicing.

Pro Tip

Add a teaspoon of banana extract and ½ cup of walnuts for yummy banana bread.

TEASE ME

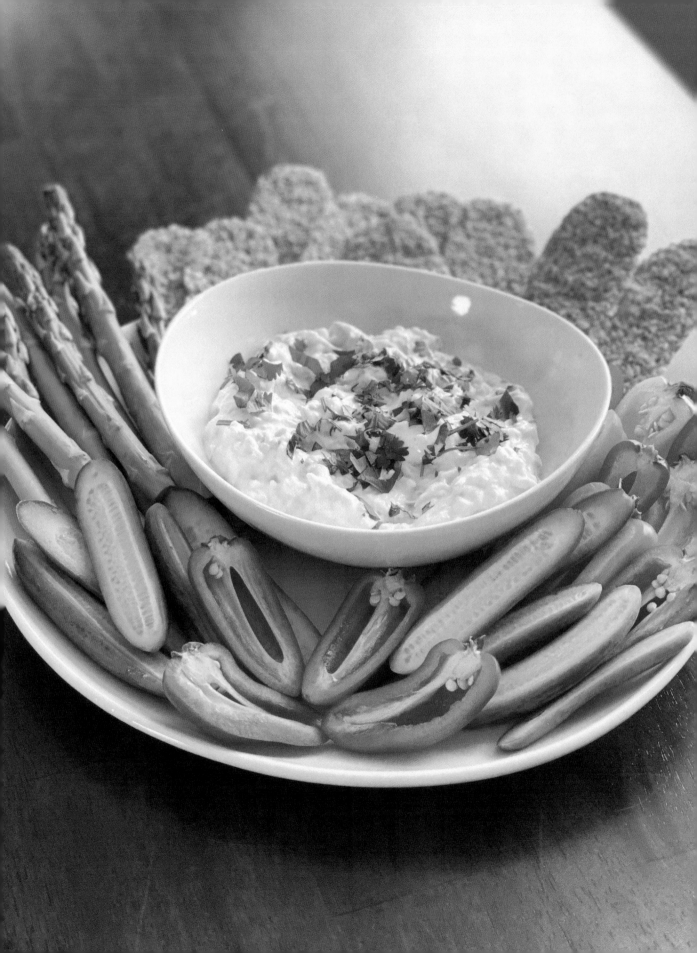

SPINACH, ARTICHOKE, AND JALAPEÑO DIP

Ingredients

- 8 ounces cream cheese, softened
- 1 cup sour cream
- ½ cup heavy whipping cream
- ¾ cup mozzarella cheese (reserve ¼ cup for topping)
- 1½ cups grated parmesan cheese (reserve 1/2 cup for topping)
- 14-ounce jar artichoke hearts
- 4-ounce can diced jalapeños
- 10 ounces frozen spinach
- 1 tablespoon minced garlic
- 1 teaspoon salt
- ½ teaspoon pepper

Directions

1. Preheat oven to 375°F.
2. In a saucepan over medium heat, whisk cream cheese, sour cream, and heavy cream together until combined.
3. Add salt, pepper, 1 cup of parmesan, and ½ cup of mozzarella cheese. Stir until cheese is melted.
4. Bring to a simmer and add chopped artichokes, thawed and drained spinach, jalapeños, and garlic.
5. Mix well and allow to heat through.
6. Pour mixture in a shallow baking dish, top with remaining mozzarella and parmesan cheese and bake for 15-20 minutes or until cheese is golden and bubbly.

TEASE ME

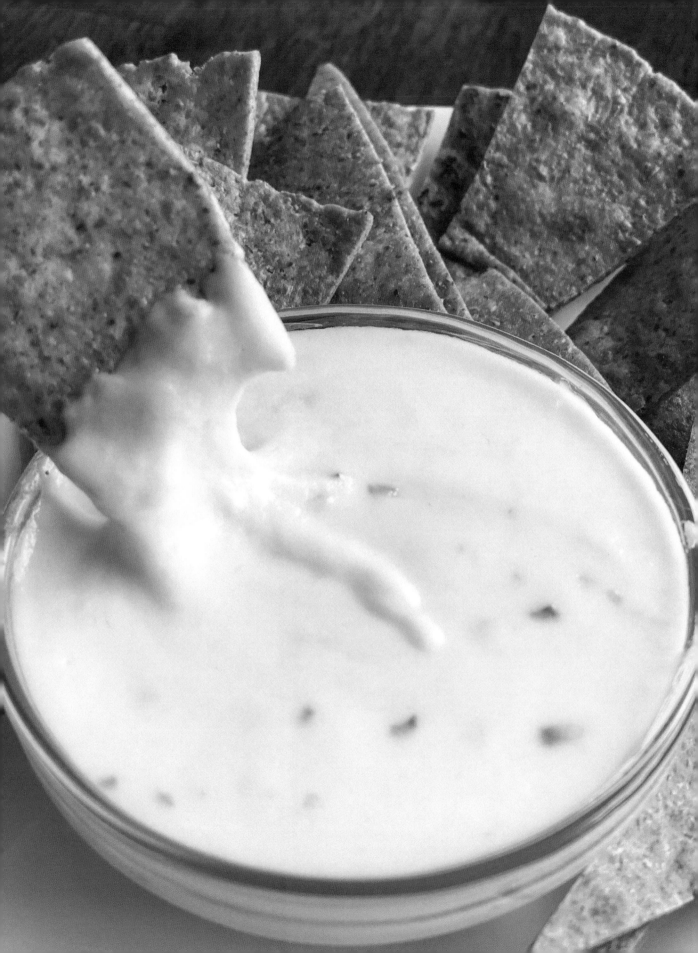

Prep Time: 3 minutes
Cook Time: 4 minutes
Yield: 10 servings
(2 tablespoons each)

QUESO BLANCO

Ingredients

1 cup shredded pepper jack cheese
½ cup heavy whipping cream
¼ cup sour cream
1 teaspoon salt
½ teaspoon pepper

Directions

1. Mix all ingredients in a microwave-safe bowl. Heat in 30-second intervals until melted and well combined.
2. Serve with pork rinds, veggies, or low-carb tortillas crisped in the oven.

Pro Tip

Add 2 ounces of diced green chilies and a ½ can of hot Ro-Tel tomatoes for an extra kick if you like to keep things spicy!

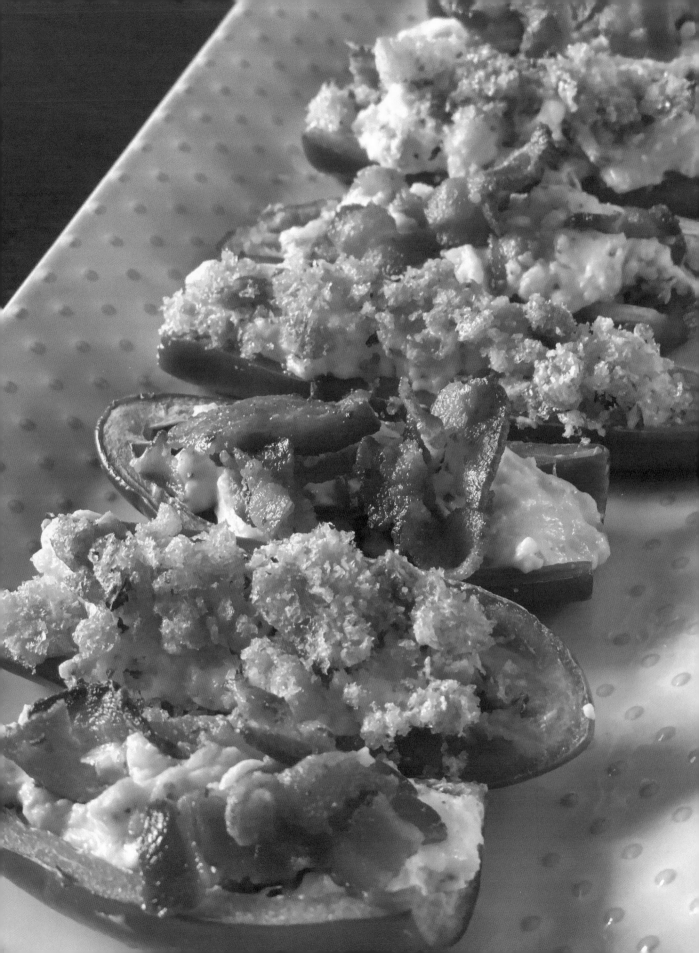

JALAPEÑO POPPERS

Ingredients

Directions

6 jalapeño peppers
3 ounces cream cheese, softened
½ teaspoon garlic powder
2 ounces shredded sharp cheddar cheese

TOPPINGS

3 slices bacon, pan-fried and crumbled
¼ cup pork rinds, crushed
2 tablespoons parmesan cheese, grated
1 teaspoon Italian seasoning
2 tablespoons butter, melted

1. Preheat oven to 400°F and line a baking sheet with parchment paper.
2. Prep the jalapeños by slicing lengthwise and using a spoon to clean out seeds and membranes.
3. In a small mixing bowl, combine the cream cheese, garlic powder, and sharp cheddar cheese.
4. In a separate bowl, stir together crushed pork rinds, parmesan cheese, Italian seasoning, and melted butter.
5. Fill jalapeños with cheese mixture. At this point, you can top with the bacon and/or the pork rind crumb mixture.
6. Place jalapeños on the baking sheet and bake for 18-23 minutes or until golden.
7. Remove from oven and allow to cool for 5 minutes before serving.Try dipping these into some ranch*.

TEASE ME

*Ranch recipe on page 191.

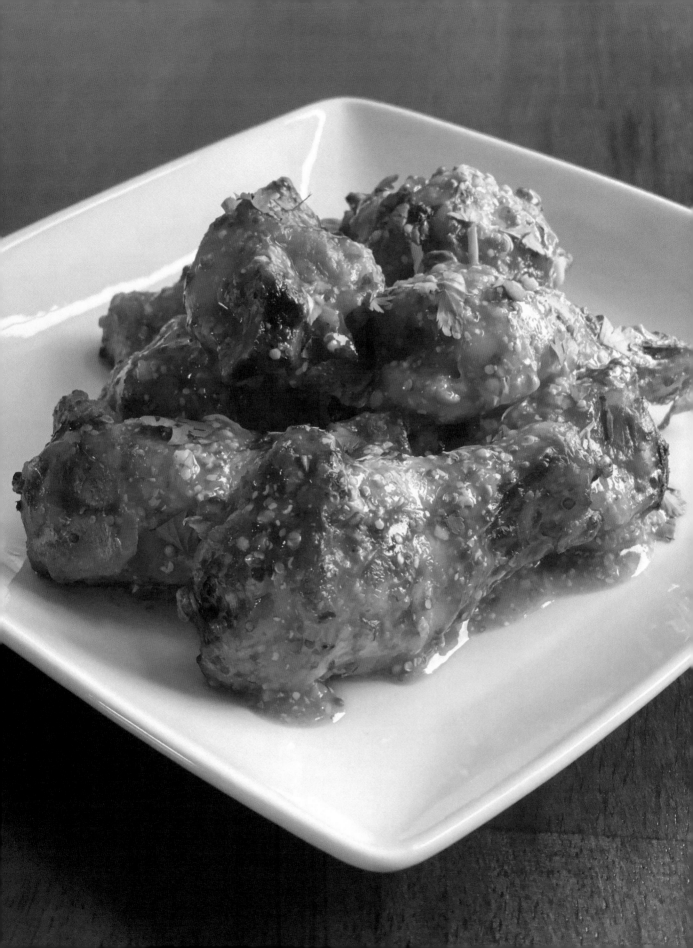

MAPLE MUSTARD WINGS

Ingredients

24 chicken wings
2 tablespoons melted butter
1 teaspoon salt
½ teaspoon pepper
½ cup sugar-free maple pancake syrup
3 teaspoons Dijon mustard
2 tablespoons soy sauce or coconut aminos
1 teaspoon minced garlic
2 teaspoons Sriracha sauce
1 teaspoon red pepper flakes
Scallions for garnish

Directions

1. Preheat oven to 400°F and line baking sheet with parchment paper.
2. In a medium mixing bowl, whisk together melted butter, salt, pepper, sugar-free maple syrup, Dijon mustard, soy sauce, garlic, Sriracha sauce, and red pepper flakes.
3. In a large bowl, pour half of the sauce over the wings and toss until well coated.
4. Place wings on baking sheet and bake for 45 mins, flipping half was through.
5. Brush with remaining sauce and cook an additional 15 minutes.
6. Garnish with scallions and serve hot.

Pro Tip

Instead of the oven, use an air fryer and cook the wings naked, with no sauce, at 400°F for 12 minutes. Flip, and cook for an additional 12 minutes until golden. Remove from air fryer and coat with sauce. If you want crispier wings, return to air fryer and cook for an additional 5 minutes.

TEASE ME

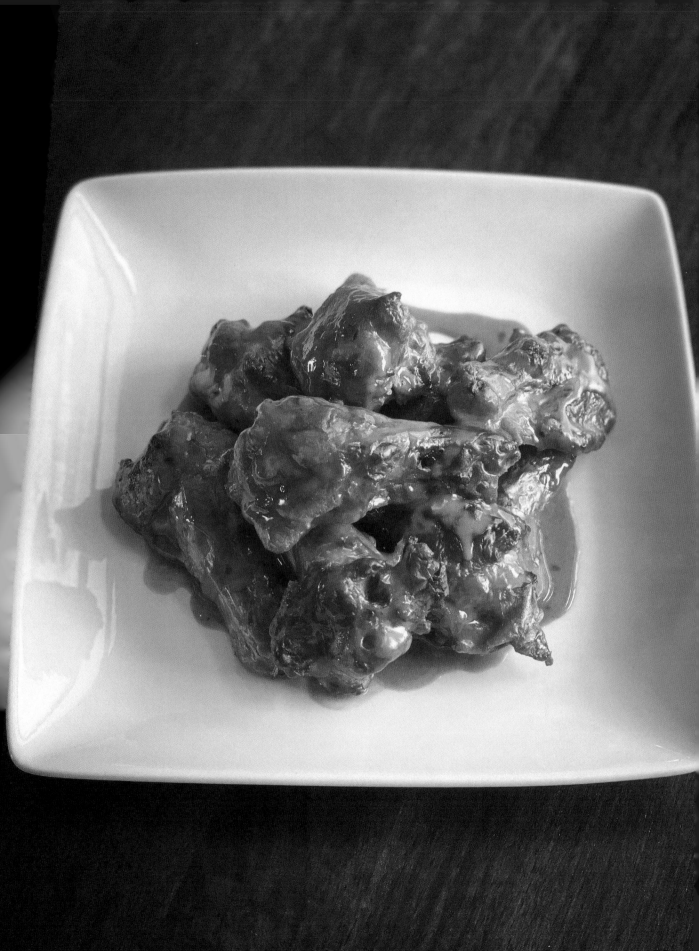

Prep Time: 15 minutes
Cook Time: 45 minutes
Yield: 6 servings

STICKY PEANUT BUTTER & JELLY WINGS

Ingredients

24 chicken wings
12-ounce jar sugar-free grape jelly
½ cup natural creamy peanut butter
¼ cup rice wine vinegar
½ teaspoon salt
¼ teaspoon pepper
½ teaspoon chili powder
Juice of half a lemon

Directions

1. Preheat oven to 400°F and line a baking sheet with parchment paper.
2. In a large mixing bowl, stir together the jelly, peanut butter, rice wine vinegar, salt, pepper, chili powder, and lemon juice.
3. Using half of the marinade, coat the chicken wings and chill for 1 hour up to 24 hours.
4. Place marinated wings on the baking sheet.
5. Bake for 45 minutes, flipping half way through and basting wings with marinade before returning to the oven.
6. Heat the remaining marinade in a saucepan on medium heat. When wings are golden and crispy, pull from oven and coat in remaining marinade sauce.

Pro Tip

Instead of the oven, use an air fryer and cook the wings naked, with no sauce, at 400°F for 12 minutes. Flip, and cook for an additional 12 minutes until golden. Remove from air fryer and coat with sauce. If you want crispier wings, return to air fryer and cook for an additional 5 minutes.

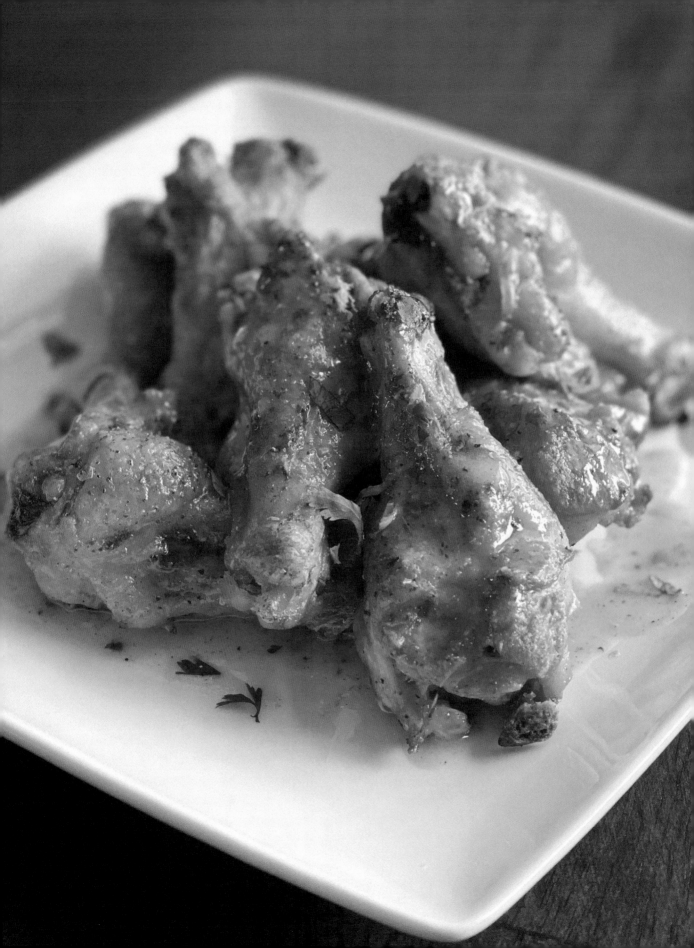

GARLICY LEMON PEPPER WINGS

Ingredients

24 chicken wings
¾ cup butter
1 teaspoon salt
½ teaspoon pepper
3 tablespoons lemon pepper seasoning
1 teaspoon minced garlic
Juice and zest of 1 large lemon
2 tablespoons parmesan cheese
1 tablespoon fresh parsley for garnish

Directions

1. Preheat oven to 400°F and line a baking sheet with parchment paper.
2. Place wings on a baking sheet and bake for 45 minutes, flipping halfway through.
3. While the wings cook, melt the butter in the microwave. Stir in salt, pepper, lemon pepper, garlic, zest and juice of 1 lemon and set aside.
4. Once wings are done, place them in a large bowl and pour half of the butter mixture on top of the wings and toss.
5. Return wings to the baking sheet, and cook an additional 10 minutes.
6. Pour remaining butter sauce over wings and top with parmesan cheese. Garnish with fresh parsley.

TEASE ME

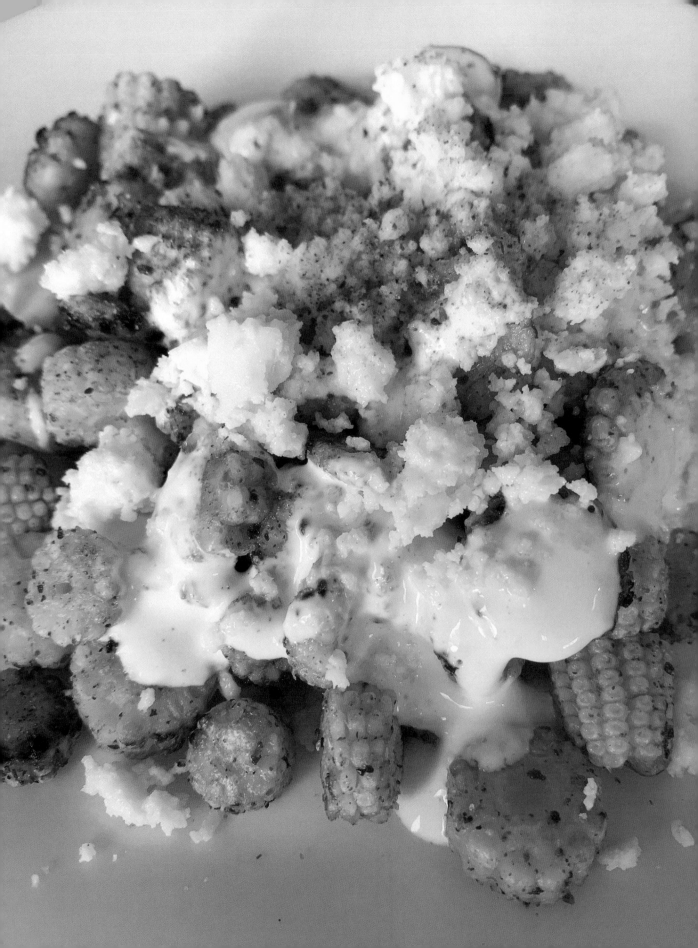

Prep Time: 5 minutes
Cook Time: 10 minutes
Yield: 4 servings

ELOTE IN A BOWL

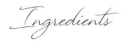

Ingredients

1 can baby corn, drained
¼ cup sour cream
¼ cup mayonnaise
2 tablespoons parmesan cheese
¼ teaspoon cumin
½ teaspoon garlic powder
½ teaspoon onion powder
1 teaspoon chili powder
Salt and pepper to taste
1 tablespoon lime juice
2 tablespoons butter
½ teaspoon cilantro

Directions

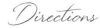

1. In a medium mixing bowl, whisk together sour cream, mayonnaise, parmesan cheese, seasonings, and lime juice. Set aside while you make the corn.
2. Melt butter in a large skillet on medium-high heat.
3. Chop the baby corn in bite-size pieces and toss into the pan. Cook until lightly golden and edges are starting to brown.
4. Remove from heat and toss corn in the sauce. Mix to coat thoroughly.
5. Top with extra parmesan cheese, a few squeezes of lime juice, chili powder, and cilantro for garnish.

Pro Tip

Replace the parmesan cheese with cotija!

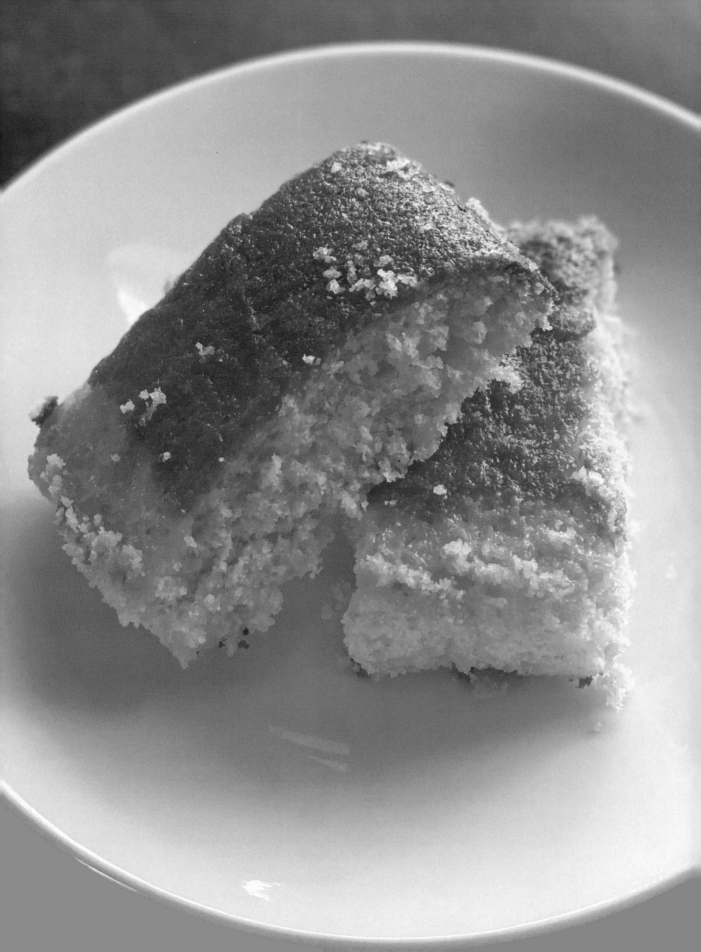

Prep Time: 10 minutes
Cook Time: 25 minutes
Yield: 6 servings

CORNBREAD

Ingredients

1 ½ cups almond flour
2 teaspoons baking powder
4 eggs
4 tablespoons butter (reserve 2 tablespoons for cast iron skillet)
1/4 can baby corn, chopped
2 tablespoons juice from baby corn
2 tablespoons sour cream
¼ cup powdered sweetener
½ teaspoon salt

Directions

1. Preheat oven to 350°F
2. In a large mixing bowl, stir together almond flour, baking powder, and powdered sweetener.
3. In a separate bowl, whisk eggs, 2 tablespoons of melted butter, corn juice, sour cream, and powdered sweetener.
4. Slowly add wet ingredients into the dry ingredients, being careful to not over mix. Gently, fold in chopped baby corn
5. Melt the remaining 2 tablespoons of butter in a cast-iron skillet to coat the pan. Pour batter in a cast-iron skillet and bake for 20-25 minutes or until a toothpick comes out clean.
6. Allow cornbread to rest and cool for at least 10 minutes. Slice and top with butter.

Pro Tip

Kick up the heat by adding diced jalapeños to the batter.

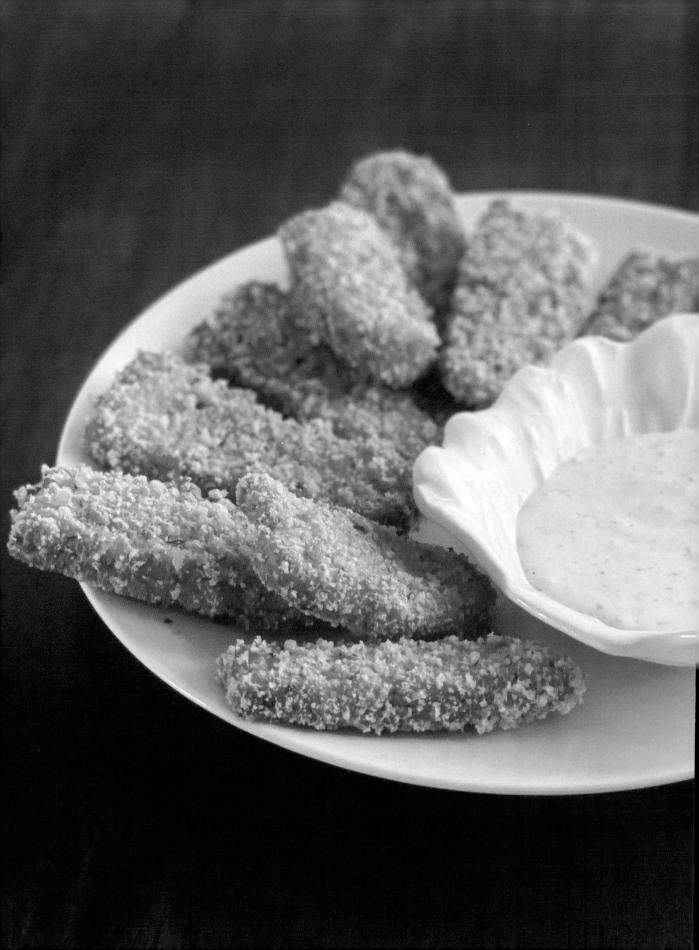

Prep Time: 5 minutes
Cook Time: 10 minutes
Yield: 8 servings

RIDE 'EM COWBOY PICKLES

Ingredients

1 cup thick-sliced pickles
½ cup almond flour
1 egg
½ cup half & half
1 cup crushed pork rinds
½ cup parmesan cheese
2 teaspoons seasoning salt
1 teaspoon Worcestershire sauce
¼ cup oil for frying

Directions

1. Heat oil in a medium pan on medium-high heat.
2. Set up a three-bowl dredging station. In first bowl, whisk egg, half & half, and Worcestershire sauce. In another bowl, mix together almond flour and 2 teaspoons of seasoning salt. For the last bowl, stir together crushed pork rinds and parmesan cheese.
3. Take sliced pickles and dredge in this order: first dip in the egg mixture, then the almond flour mixture, and lastly, dip in the pork rind mixture.
4. Shallow-fry pickles in oil until golden brown and crispy.
5. Place on paper towels to absorb excess oil and sprinkle with salt while hot. Serve with homemade ranch*.

TEASE ME

*Ranch recipe on page 191.

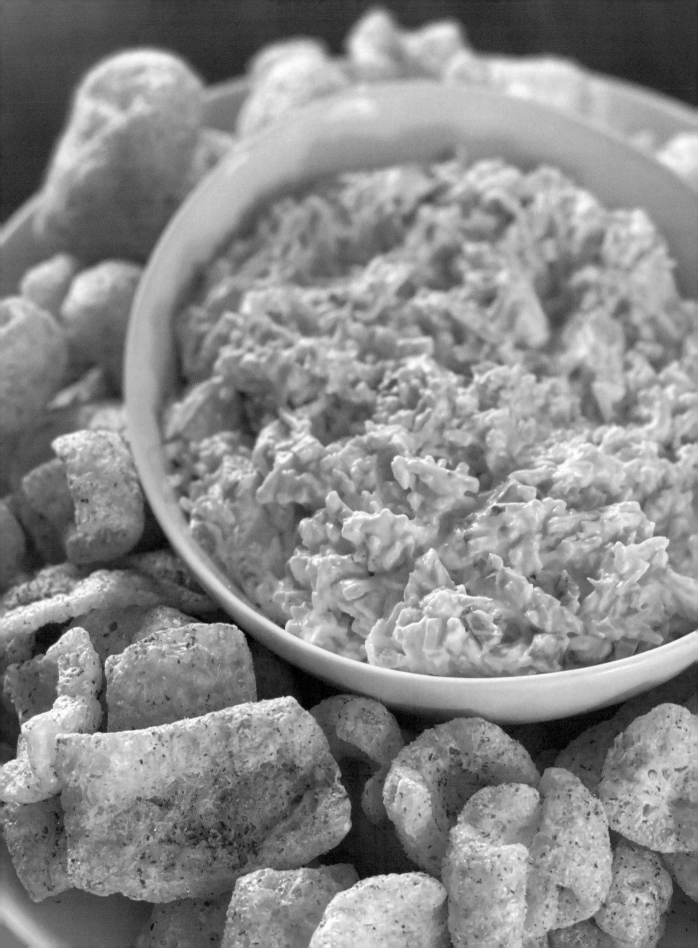

Prep Time: 10 minutes
Cook Time: 0 minutes
Yield: 14 servings
(2 tablespoons each)

JALAPEÑO PIMENTO CHEESE

Ingredients

1 pound cheddar cheese, shredded
4-ounce jar pimentos
2 chopped jalapeños
4 ounces cream cheese, softened
½ cup mayonnaise
1 tablespoon onion, grated
½ teaspoon black pepper
1 teaspoon garlic powder
1 teaspoon salt
½ teaspoon pepper

Directions

1. Prep your jalapeños by cutting them in half lengthwise, removing the ribs and seeds if you do not want your cheese to be too spicy, and then dice.
2. In a medium mixing bowl, stir jalapeños together with the remainder of the ingredients.
3. Chill in the refrigerator for an hour before serving. Enjoy as a dip or top of your favorite meats and veggies.

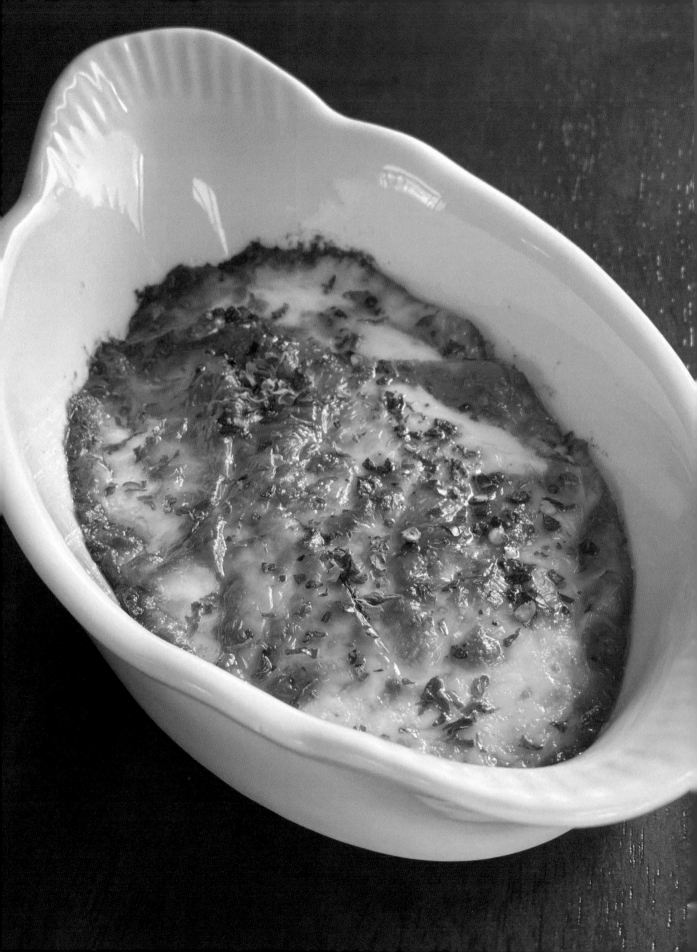

Prep Time: 3 minutes
Cook Time: 10 minutes
Yield: 1 serving

OVEN-BAKED CHEESE

Ingredients

¾ cup shredded mozzarella cheese
½ teaspoon dried parsley
½ teaspoon red pepper flakes

Directions

1. Preheat oven to 400°F.
2. Place shredded cheese in an oven safe dish. Top with seasonings.
3. Bake for 8-10 minuets.

Pro Tip

Instead of using the oven, try cooking in the air fryer at 400°F for 6-7 minutes.

TEASE ME

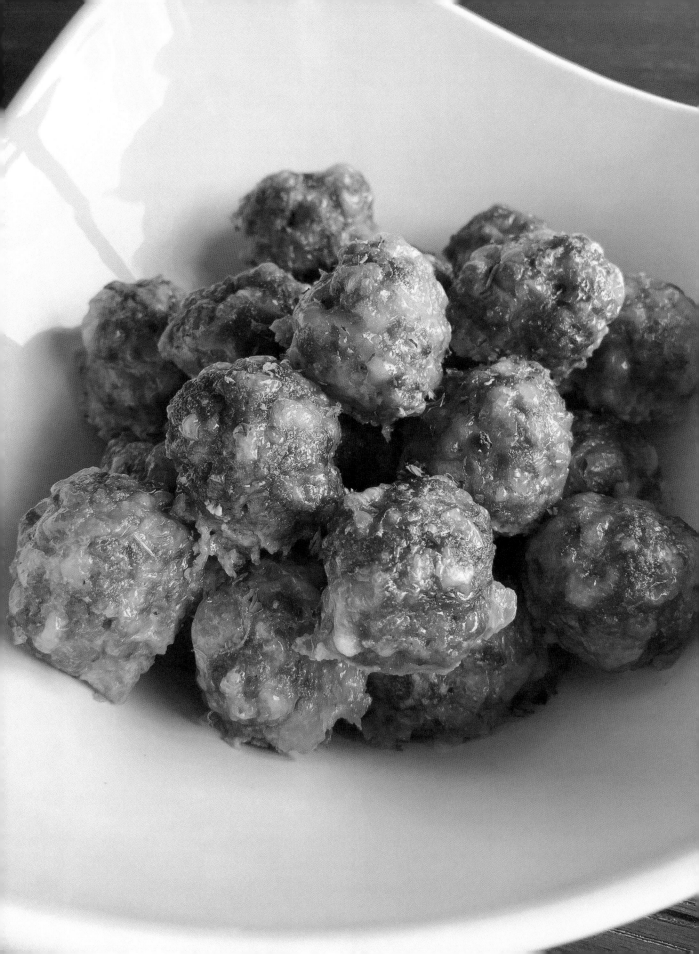

Prep Time: 10 minutes
Cook Time: 20 minutes
Yield: 6 servings

PARTY MEATBALLS

Ingredients

1 pound ground beef
1 egg
½ cup parmesan cheese
½ cup mozzarella cheese, shredded
¼ cup sharp cheddar cheese, shredded
1 tablespoon minced garlic
1 teaspoon black pepper
½ teaspoon salt

Directions

1. Preheat oven to 400°F and line baking sheet with parchment paper.
2. In a large mixing bowl, combine all ingredients and knead together until combined.
3. Roll mixture into evenly-sized balls and place on baking sheet.
4. Bake for 18-20 minutes.

TEASE ME

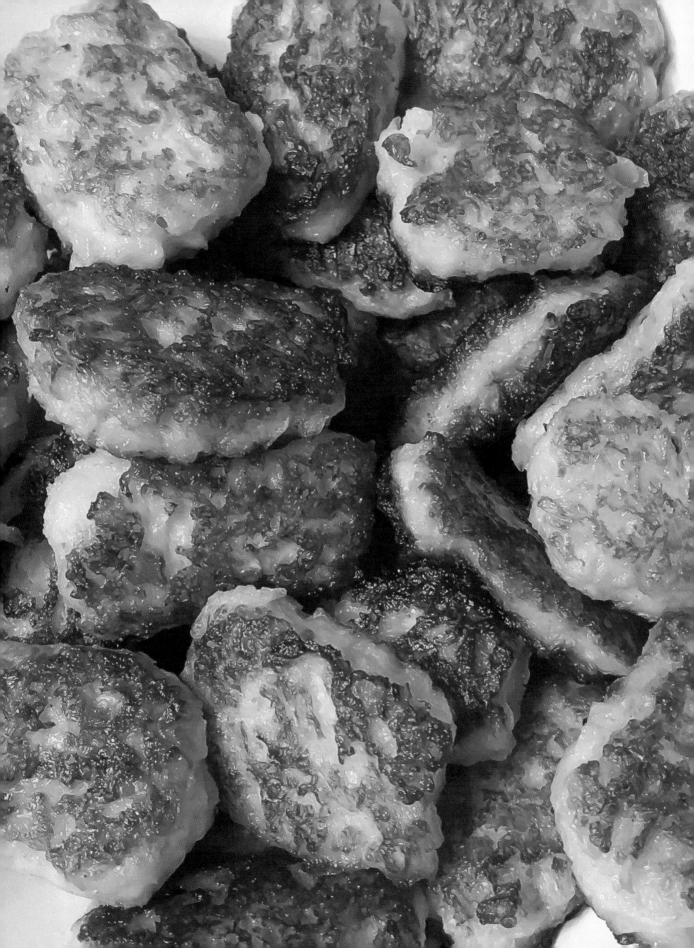

Prep Time: 10 minutes
Cook Time: 15 minutes
Yield: 6 servings

Ingredients

2 bags frozen riced cauliflower
  (10 ounces each)
¼ cup oil, divided
1 egg
1 ½ cups mozzarella cheese, shredded
1 teaspoon minced garlic
¾ teaspoon salt

FAUX-TATO TOTS

Directions

1. Using a large mixing bowl, whisk the egg and mix in the mozzarella cheese, garlic, and salt.
2. In a large skillet, stir-fry the frozen cauliflower in 2 tablespoons of oil until tender and lightly golden with no moisture left in pan. While still hot, stir the cauliflower into the bowl. This will melt the cheese and make the mixture sticky.
3. Using your hands, roll mixture into evenly-sized tots and gently flatten to form a coin.
4. Heat remaining oil in a skillet over medium heat. Add tots to the oil in a single layer, spaced apart, and fry for about 2 minutes until golden. Flip, and fry an additional 2 minutes before transferring to a paper towel to drain excess oil.

TEASE ME

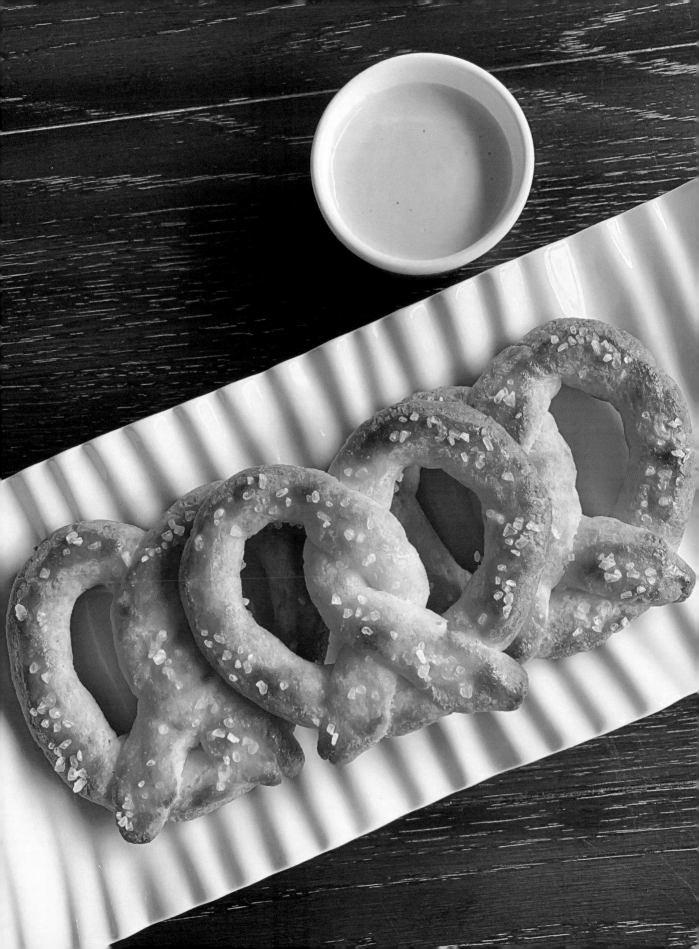

Prep Time: 10 minutes
Cook Time: 15 minutes
Yield: 6 servings

JUMBO SOFT PRETZELS

Ingredients

2 cups shredded mozzarella cheese
2 ounces cream cheese
1 egg
1 tablespoon baking powder
1 teaspoon garlic powder
1 teaspoon onion powder
1 cup almond flour
Coarse sea salt for topping

Directions

1. Preheat oven to 425°F and line a baking sheet with parchment paper.
2. In a microwave-safe bowl, melt mozzarella and cream cheese in 30-second intervals, stirring in between until melted. This will take around 1 minute.
3. Add remaining ingredients. Mix with a fork or knead with your hands until thoroughly combined. If dough is super sticky, add a little more almond flour.
4. Divide dough into 6 parts, roll each into a long rope, and fold into a pretzel shape. Top with coarse salt.
5. Place onto baking sheet and bake for 12-15 minutes or until lightly golden and serve with beer cheese*.

Pro Tip

Instead of salt, sprinkle a little granular sweetener mixed with ground cinnamon over the top for a sweet treat.

*Beer cheese recipe on page 187.

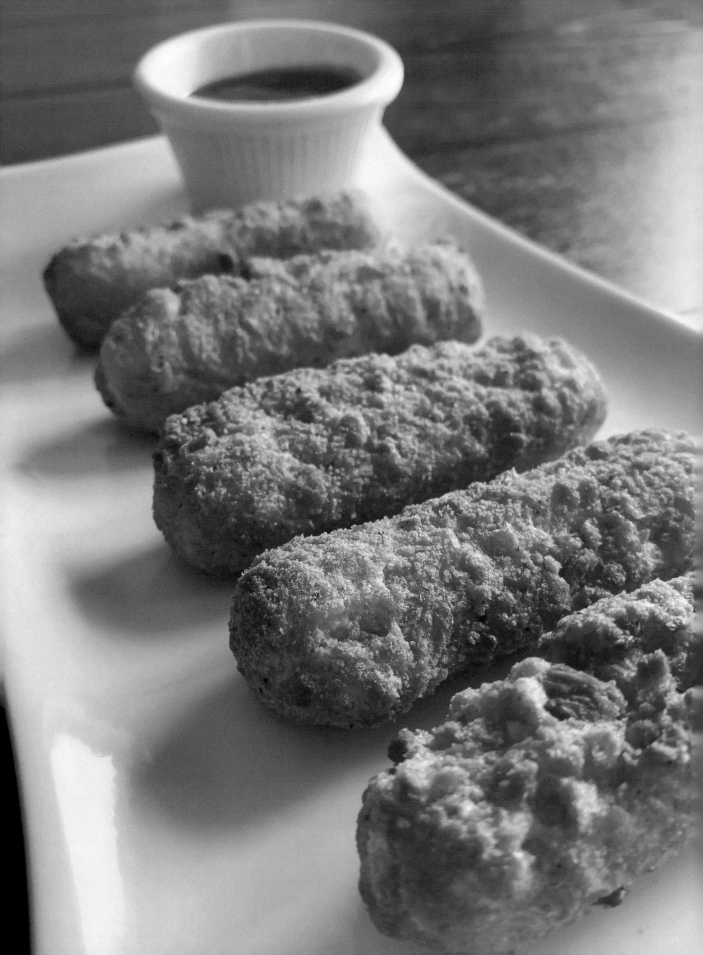

Prep Time: 5 minutes
Cook Time: 10 minutes
Yield: 6 servings

FRIED MOZZARELLA STICKS

Ingredients

6 mozzarella cheese sticks cut in half
2 eggs, lightly beaten
1 cup crushed pork rinds
1 tablespoon Italian seasoning
½ cup unflavored protein powder
1 teaspoon salt
½ teaspoon pepper
Avocado oil for frying

Directions

1. Set up a 3-bowl dredging station. For the first bowl mix together protein powder, salt, and pepper. In the second bowl, add in the beaten eggs. Mix together the crushed pork rinds and Italian season in the third bowl.
2. Dip mozzarella stick in first station and shake off extra protein powder. Then, dip the cheese in the egg before rolling in the pork rinds.
3. Heat oil in a large skillet on medium-high heat and shallow fry each stick until golden
4. Serve with ranch* or your favorite no-sugar-added marinara sauce.

*Ranch recipe on page 191.

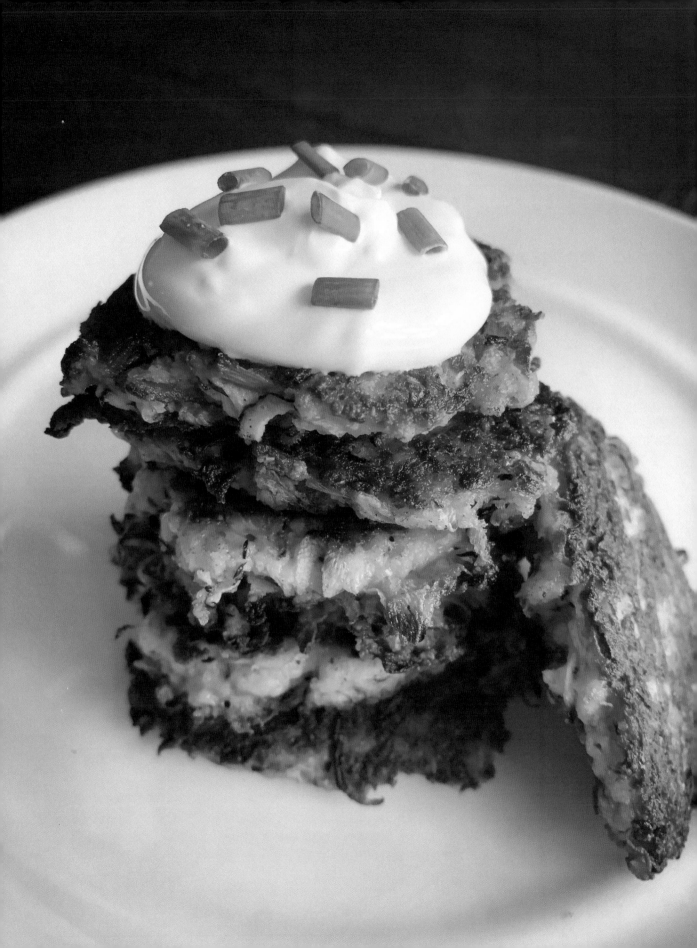

Prep Time: 25 minutes
Cook Time: 10 minutes
Yield: 4 servings

ZUCCHINI FRITTERS

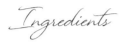

Ingredients

2 medium zucchini, grated (about 2 cups)
2 slices bacon
⅓ cup almond flour
3 green onion sprigs, chopped
1 teaspoon minced garlic
¼ cup cheddar cheese, shredded
Salt and pepper to taste

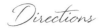

Directions

1. Using a cheese grater, shred the zucchini. Sprinkle with salt and stir before placing in a colander in the sink to drain. Let sit for 20 minutes. To further drain the liquid, place in a cheesecloth or dishtowel and squeeze.
2. In a large skillet, fry the bacon and then chop. (Reserve the bacon grease)
3. Using a large bowl, combine all ingredients and mix well.
4. Heat the skillet with leftover bacon grease on medium-high heat. Scoop batter out with a cookie scoop (roughly 1 tablespoon) and place in hot skillet. Gently press down with a spatula to flatten. Fry for 2 minutes or until golden, flip, and continue to fry for an additional 2 minutes. Serve with sour cream and chives.

TEASE ME

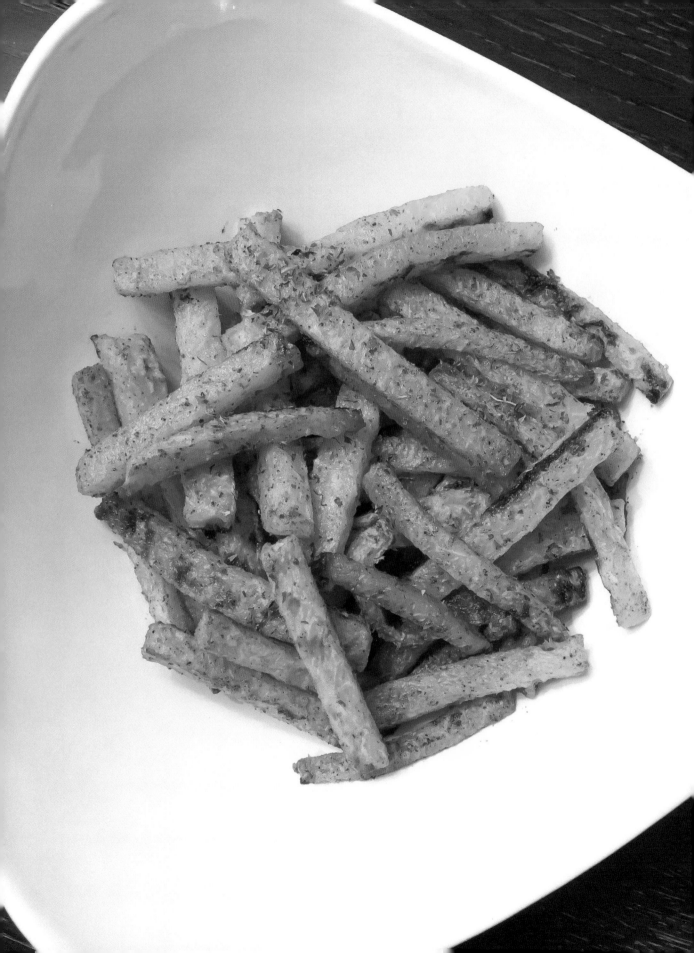

Prep Time: 15 minutes
Cook Time: 10 minutes
Yield: 4 servings

JICAMA FRIES

Ingredients

1 large jicama (around 1 pound)
1 ½ teaspoons salt
½ teaspoon ground turmeric
¼ teaspoon garlic powder
¼ teaspoon paprika
⅛ teaspoon onion powder
1 scoop unflavored protein powder
Avocado oil for frying

Directions

1. Using a vegetable peeler, peal the skin off the jicama and slice into thin matchsticks.
2. In a large pot over high heat, fill with water and add ½ teaspoon of salt. Bring to a boil before adding jicama. Cover with lid and boing for 10 minutes. Remove pot from heat and drain water.
3. Place jicama in a large mixing bowl. Add remaining 1teaspoon of salt, turmeric, garlic powder, paprika, onion powder, and protein powder. Toss with tongs until jicama is fully-coated in spices.
4. Heat avocado oil in a large pan on high. Fry jicama until golden, roughly 10 minutes. Place on paper towels to drain excess oil. While fries are hot, sprinkle with any additional seasonings. Serve with no-sugar-added ketchup.

Pro Tip

Instead of boiling jicama, you can simply microwave the jicama in a large bowl with a damp paper towel over the top for 8-10 minutes.

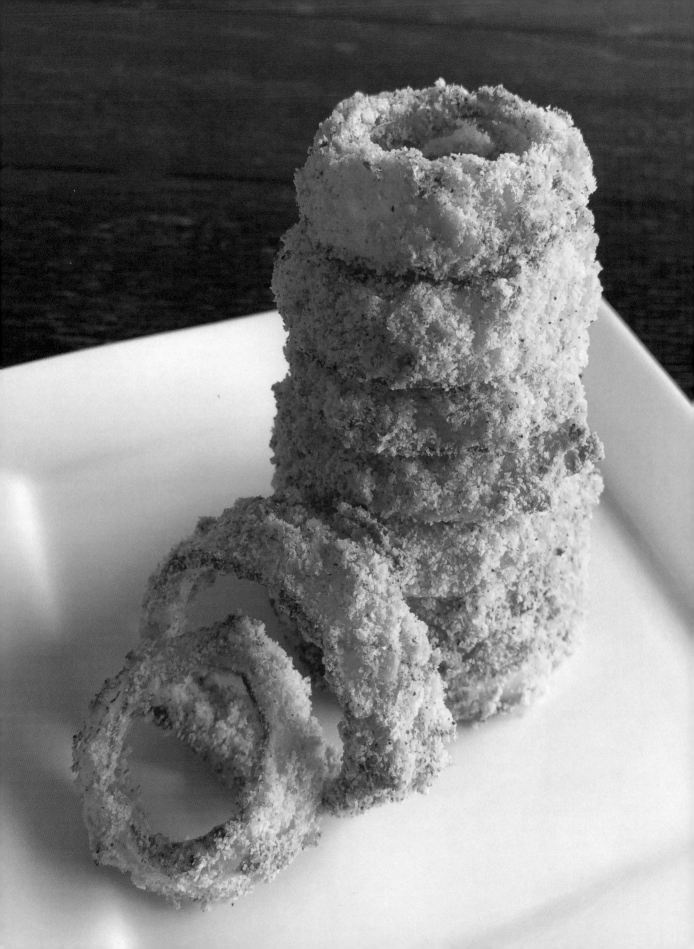

Prep Time: 15 minutes
Cook Time: 18 minutes
Yield: 4 servings

ONION RINGS

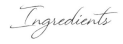

Ingredients

1 large onion cut into ½-inch thick rings
1 scoop unflavored protein powder
¼ teaspoon seasoning salt
2 eggs
1 cup pork rinds
3 tablespoons almond flour
¼ teaspoon cayenne pepper
1 teaspoon garlic powder

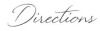

Directions

1. Preheat oven to 400°F and line a baking sheet with parchment paper.
2. Crush 1 cup of pork rinds.
3. Set up a dredging station of three shallow bowls. In bowl one, stir together unflavored protein powder and salt. For the second bowl, add two eggs and whisk. In the last bowl, mix together crushed pork rinds, almond flour, cayenne pepper, and garlic powder.
4. Dredge the onion rings in the coconut flour, then dip into the egg, and finally, place in the pork rind mixture, scooping it over the ring to fully coat it. Place rings on baking sheet and bake for 16-18 minutes or until golden and crispy.

Pro Tip

Instead of the oven, try cooking in the air fryer at 400°F for 15 minutes.

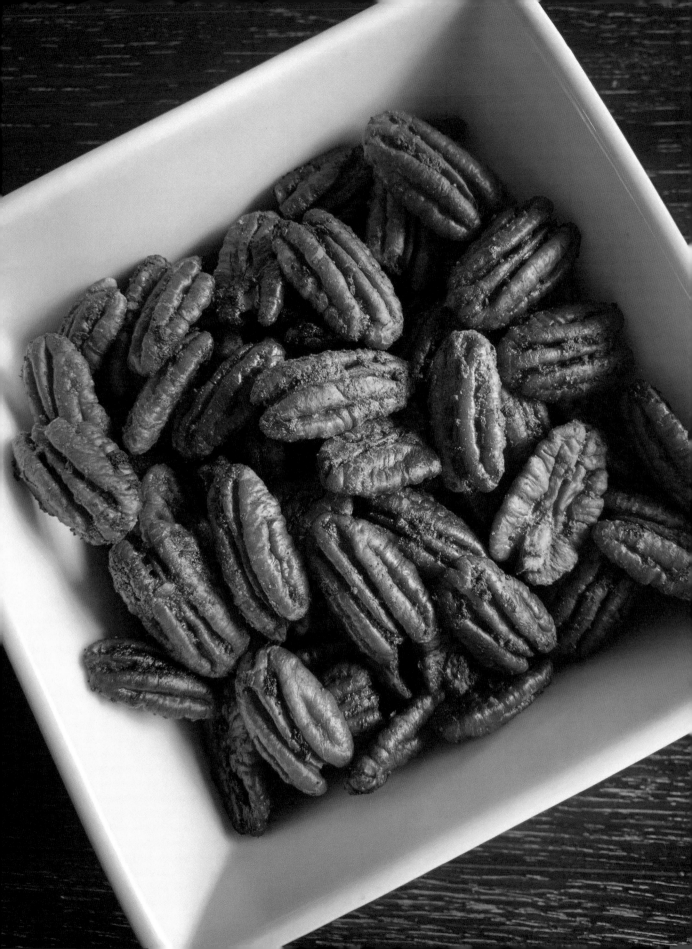

Prep Time: 10 minutes
Cook Time: 30 minutes
Yield: 8 servings
(2 ounces each)

PARTY PECANS

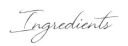

Ingredients

1 pound pecan halves
4 tablespoons butter, melted
3 tablespoons Worcestershire sauce
1 packet of spicy ranch seasoning
¾ teaspoon garlic powder
¾ teaspoon onion powder

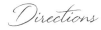

Directions

1. Preheat oven to 300°F.
2. In a large mixing bowl, mix together melted butter, Worcestershire sauce, ranch seasoning, garlic powder, and onion powder. Pour in pecans and stir until well coated.
3. Spread pecans on a baking sheet in a single layer and bake for 30 minutes, stirring every 10 minutes.
4. Allow to cool before eating.

TEASE ME

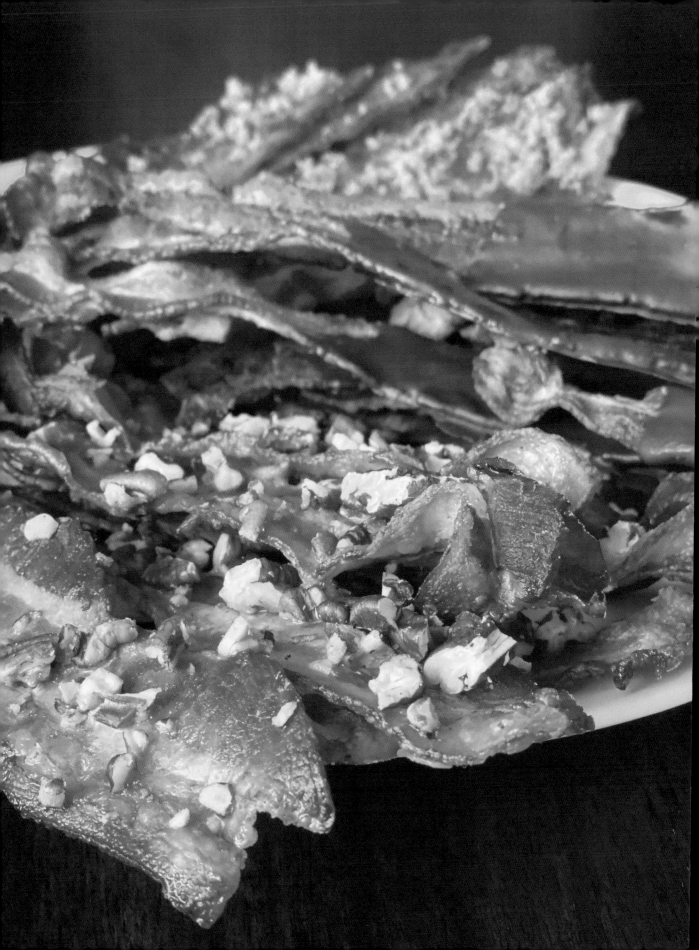

Prep Time: 5 minutes
Cook Time: 15 minutes
Yield: 12 servings

3-WAY BACON AFFAIR

CHOCOLATE DIPPED BACON

Ingredients

1 pound thick cut bacon
¾ cup no-sugar-added chocolate chips, melted
¼ cup salty peanuts, chopped

Directions

1. Preheat oven to 425°F and line a baking sheet with parchment paper
2. Arrange bacon on the baking sheet in single layer and cook for 15 minutes or until desired crispiness is achieved.
3. Remove from oven and allow to cool.
4. In a mug, melt chocolate chips in the microwave for 30 second intervals, stirring in between, until smooth.
5. Dip bacon into the chocolate and place on a wire rack. Sprinkle with chopped peanuts and allow chocolate to set.

PECAN PRALINE BACON

Ingredients

1 pound thick cut bacon
8 tablespoons butter
¾ cup Swerve brown sugar replacement
½ teaspoon vanilla extract
¼ cup heavy whipping cream
¼ cup pecans, chopped

Directions

1. Preheat oven to 425°F and line a baking sheet with parchment paper
2. Arrange bacon on the baking sheet in single layer and cook for 15 minutes or until desired crispiness is achieved.

3. Remove from oven and allow to cool.
4. In a medium sauce pot, melt butter on low heat. Add the brown sugar replacement and cook for 5-7 minutes while continuing to stir.
5. Mix in the heavy whipping cream and vanilla and cook for an additional 3-5 minutes as you stir.
6. Once mixture has thickened, add in the pecans and remove from heat.
7. Spoon mixture onto both sides of bacon and place on a wire rack to allow praline to set.

BOURBON CANDIED BACON

Ingredients

1 pound thick cut bacon
8 tablespoons butter
¾ cup Swerve brown sugar replacement
½ teaspoon vanilla extract
¼ cup heavy whipping cream
2 tablespoons bourbon

Directions

1. Preheat oven to 425°F and line a baking sheet with parchment paper
2. Arrange bacon on the baking sheet in single layer and cook for 15 minutes or until desired crispiness is achieved.
3. Remove from oven and allow to cool.
4. In a medium sauce pot on low heat, melt the butter.
5. Add in the brown sugar replacement and stir for 5-7 minutes.
6. Mix in the heavy whipping cream, vanilla, and bourbon and cook for an additional 3-4 minutes while continuing to stir.
6. When sauce has thickened, remove from heat and brush onto both sides of the bacon and place on a wire rack to set.

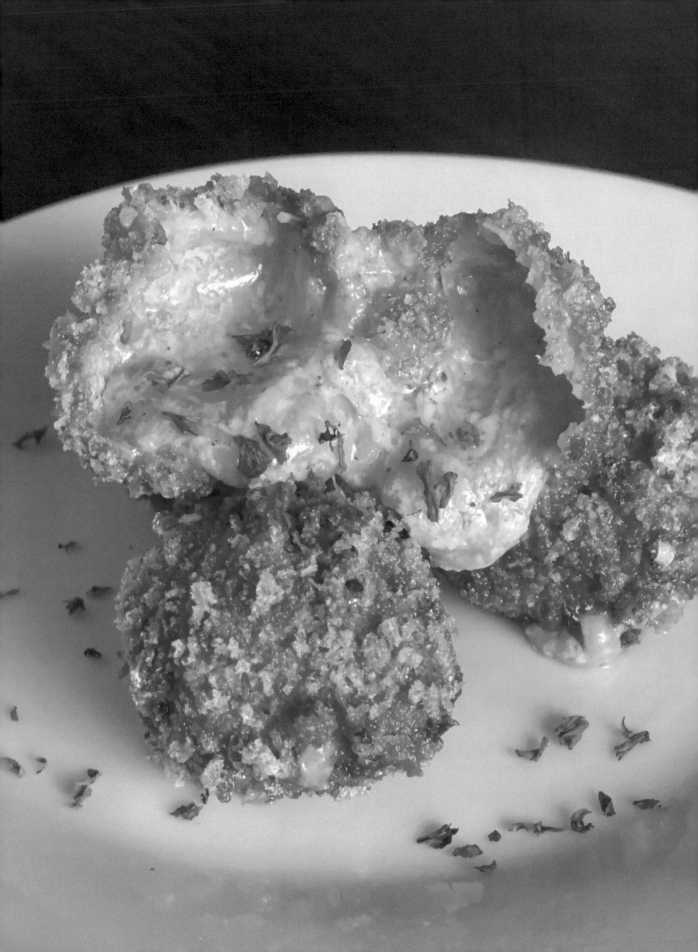

Prep Time: 45 minutes
Cook Time: 10 minutes
Yield: 8 servings

FRIED PIMENTO CHEESE BALLS

Ingredients

1 batch prepared jalapeño pimento cheese*
½ cup almond flour
1 teaspoon salt
½ teaspoon pepper
1 egg, beaten
½ cup crushed pork rinds
1 tablespoon Italian seasoning
Avocado oil for frying

Directions

1. Roll the jalapeño pimento cheese mixture into 1-inch balls and set onto a baking sheet lined with parchment paper.
2. Once all the balls are formed, place pan in refrigerator and chill for 20 minutes.
3. Set up a 3-bowl dredging station. In the first bowl, mix the almond flour, salt, and pepper. For the next bowl, add the beaten egg. Finally, in the third bowl, mix together the crushed pork rinds and Italian seasoning.
4. Remove cheese balls from refrigerator and move them through the dredging station, starting with the almond flour, moving to the egg, and, finally, the pork rinds. Place the breaded cheese balls back onto the baking sheet and return to the refrigerator to chill for an additional 20 minutes.
5. In a large pan, heat avocado oil on medium-high heat. Shallow fry cheese balls until golden brown and crispy. Serve with your favorite dipping sauce or enjoy on their own.

*Jalapeño pimento cheese recipe on page 49.

EAT

Chili

Bang Bang (Between the Sheets) Shrimp

Meatball Bake

White Chicken Enchiladas

Red Rendezvous Pork Enchiladas

Creamy Macaroni & Cheese

Coconut Shrimp with Cilantro-Lime
Cauli-Rice

Chili Cheeseburger

Chicken Satay with Peanut Sauce

Pesto Pizza

M E

BBQ Chicken pizza

Nutty Hawaiian Pizza

Chili Cheese Dog

Zucchini Au Gratin

Pigs in a Blanket

Chicken 'n Waffles

Crab Cakes

Crispy Cheese Shell Tacos

Chicken Parmesan

Buffalo Chicken Patties

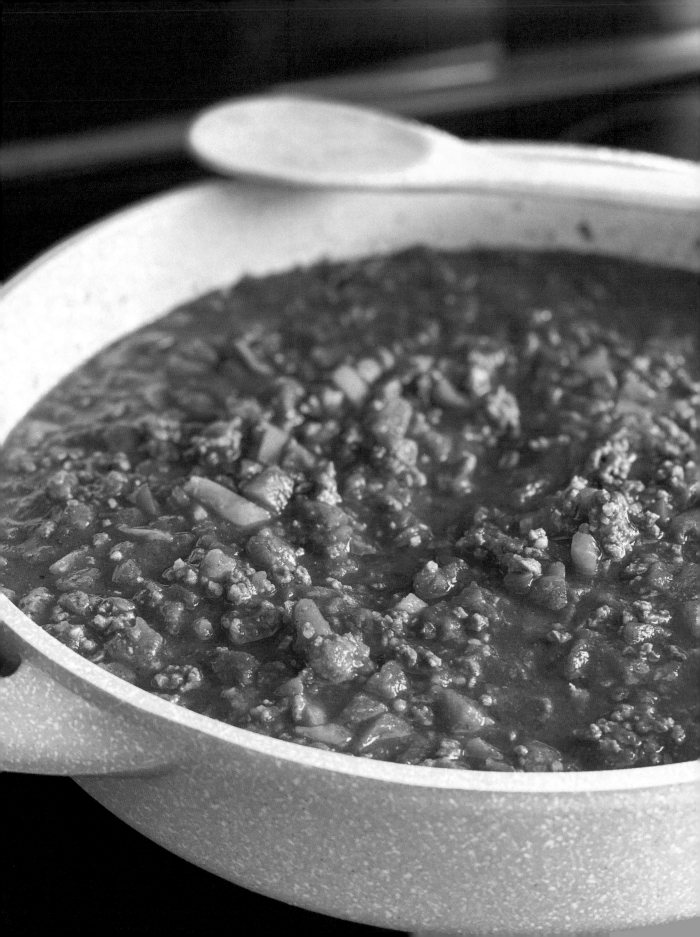

Prep Time: 20 minutes
Cook Time: 30 minutes
Yield: 12 servings

CHILI

Ingredients

2 pounds ground beef

1 pound ground Italian sausage

6 slices bacon

1 tablespoon butter

1 28-ounce can crushed tomatoes

2 15-ounce cans fire roasted tomatoes

½ cup yellow onion, chopped

1 green bell pepper, diced

½ red bell pepper, diced

1 tablespoon minced garlic

1 tablespoon cumin

2 tablespoons taco seasoning*

1 tablespoon garlic powder

1 tablespoon onion powder

1 teaspoon salt

½ teaspoon pepper

2 teaspoons chili powder

1 teaspoon red pepper flakes (optional)

Directions

1. Using a large stockpot or Dutch oven, cook bacon until crispy and drain on a paper towel.
6. Add 1 tablespoon butter to the bacon grease and melt.
7. Add chopped onion and bell peppers and cook for 3-4 minutes until softened. Add minced garlic and cook for another minute, careful not to burn.
8. Cook the beef and sausage in the pot. Do not drain
9. Mix in the seasonings and stir to combine. Add in the cans of tomatoes with the juice and simmer on medium-low heat for approximately 30 minutes while stirring occasionally. The chili will thicken as it cooks.
10. Serve hot with your favorite toppings.

*Taco seasoning recipe on page 181.

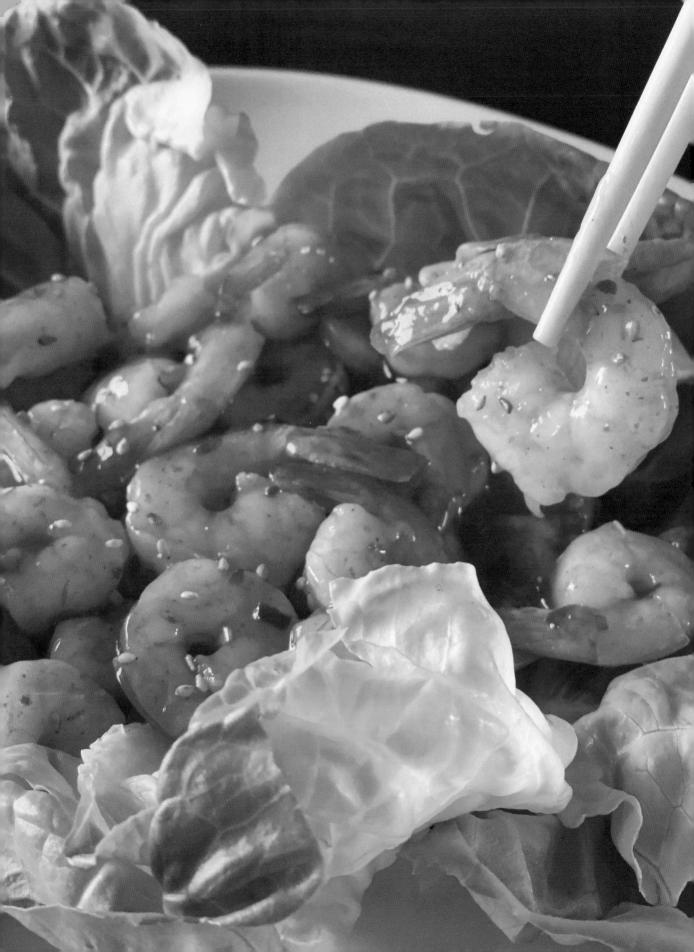

BANG BANG (BETWEEN THE SHEETS) SHRIMP

Ingredients

1 pound shrimp

3 tablespoons butter

1 shallot, finely chopped

2 tablespoons minced garlic

2 tablespoons sriracha sauce

3 tablespoons sugar-free orange marmalade

BANG BANG DIPPING SAUCE

½ cup rice wine vinegar

½ cup water

½ cup granular sweetener

3 teaspoons red pepper flakes

1 teaspoon garlic powder

½ teaspoon salt

½ teaspoon xanthan gum

Directions

1. In a large skillet, melt butter on high heat. Add shallots and garlic and cook for 2 minutes until shallots soften.
2. Stir in sriracha sauce and marmalade and simmer until the sauce thickens into a glaze.
3. Add shrimp and cook through.
4. Serve over cauliflower rice or vegetables of your choice.
5. For the dipping sauce, add all the ingredients to a medium saucepan, except the xanthan gum, and bring to a boil.
6. Boil for 5 minutes while stirring to reduce mixture.
7. Remove from heat and stir in xanthan gum.
8. Allow mixture to thicken as it cools.

Pro Tip

Use pre-cooked shrimp for a faster cooking time.

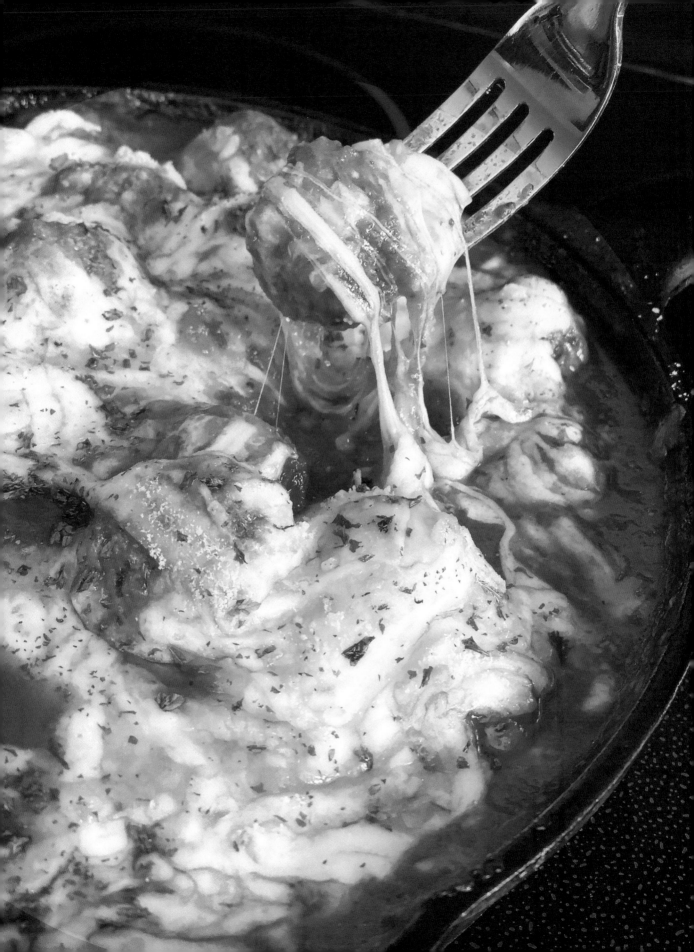

Prep Time: 10 minutes
Cook Time: 30 minutes
Yield: 4 servings

MEATBALL BAKE

Ingredients

½ pound ground beef

½ pound Italian sausage

¾ cup parmesan cheese (reserve a ¼ cup for topping)

1 egg, lightly beaten

1 teaspoon garlic powder

1 teaspoon onion powder

1 tablespoon dried parsley

½ cup crushed pork rinds

1 jar of Rao's no-sugar-added marinara sauce

¾ cup mozzarella cheese, shredded

Directions

1. Preheat oven to 375°F and line a baking sheet with parchment paper.
2. Using your hands, combine ground beef, Italian sausage, parmesan cheese, egg, garlic powder, onion powder, parsley, and crushed pork rinds.
3. Roll mixture into evenly-sized balls, place on the baking sheet and bake for 10 minutes.
4. Remove meatballs from oven and set aside.
5. Grease an 8x8 baking dish.
6. Pour half the jar of marinara sauce into the baking dish. Add the meatballs and pour in the remaining sauce.
7. Top with parmesan cheese and mozzarella cheese.
8. Bake an additional 10 to 20 minutes. Garnish with fresh parsley and enjoy on its own or with your favorite pasta alternative.

EAT ME

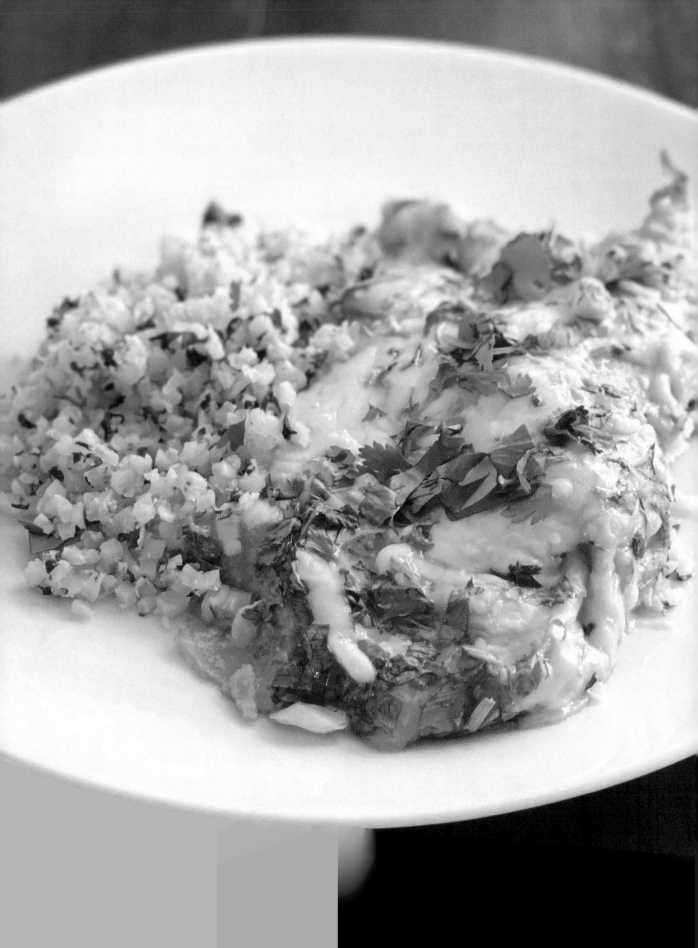

Prep Time: 15 minutes
Cook Time: 25 minutes
Yield: 4 servings

WHITE CHICKEN ENCHILADAS

Ingredients

- 1 whole rotisserie chicken, shredded
- ½ cup sour cream
- 2 cups mozzarella cheese, shredded (reserve 1 cup for topping)
- 1 teaspoon garlic powder
- 1 teaspoon onion powder
- 1 teaspoon salt
- ½ teaspoon pepper
- 1 10-ounce can green enchilada sauce
- 1 package low-carb tortillas
- Fresh cilantro for garnish

Directions

1. Preheat oven to 350°F.
2. Combine shredded chicken, sour cream, 1 cup of mozzarella cheese, garlic powder, onion powder, salt, and pepper in a large mixing bowl and set aside.
3. Heat green enchilada sauce in a medium skillet.
4. Dip tortillas in green enchilada sauce and coat both sides and then stuff with chicken mixture before rolling up.
5. Line enchiladas in a 9x13 baking dish and pour remaining green enchilada sauce over the top. Add 1 cup of mozzarella cheese and bake for 20-25 minutes until cheese is golden and bubbly.
6. Garnish with fresh cilantro and enjoy.

Pro Tip

Serve with a side of cilantro-lime cauli-rice*.

*Cilantro-lime cauli-rice recipe on page 87.

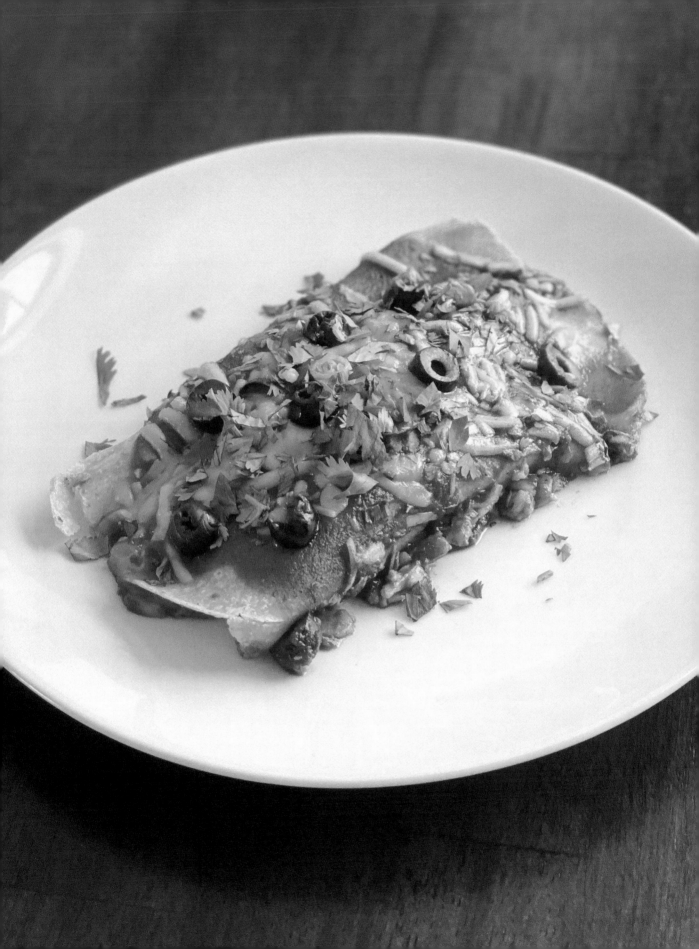

Prep Time: 15 minutes
Cook Time: 25 minutes
Yield: 4 servings

RED RENDEZVOUS PORK ENCHILADAS

Ingredients

- 1 15-ounce package of precooked pulled pork, no sauce
- 1 cup sharp cheddar cheese, shredded (reserve ½ cup for topping)
- 1 teaspoon garlic powder
- 1 teaspoon onion powder
- 1 teaspoon salt
- ½ teaspoon pepper
- 2 10-ounce cans red enchilada sauce
- 1 package low-carb tortillas
- 2 tablespoons black olives, sliced
- 2 tablespoons red onions, diced
- 2 tablespoons fresh cilantro for garnish

Directions

1. Preheat oven to 350°F.
2. Using a large mixing bowl, add pulled pork, ¾ cup red sauce, ½ cup sharp cheddar cheese, and seasonings.
3. In a medium skillet, heat ½ cup of enchilada sauce until warm. Dip tortilla in sauce and coat both sides. Fill tortillas with the pork mixture and roll up. Line enchiladas in a 9x13 baking dish.
4. Pour ½ cup of enchilada sauce over the top and sprinkle on the remaining cheese. Add olives and onions and bake for 20-25 minutes until cheese is golden and bubbly.

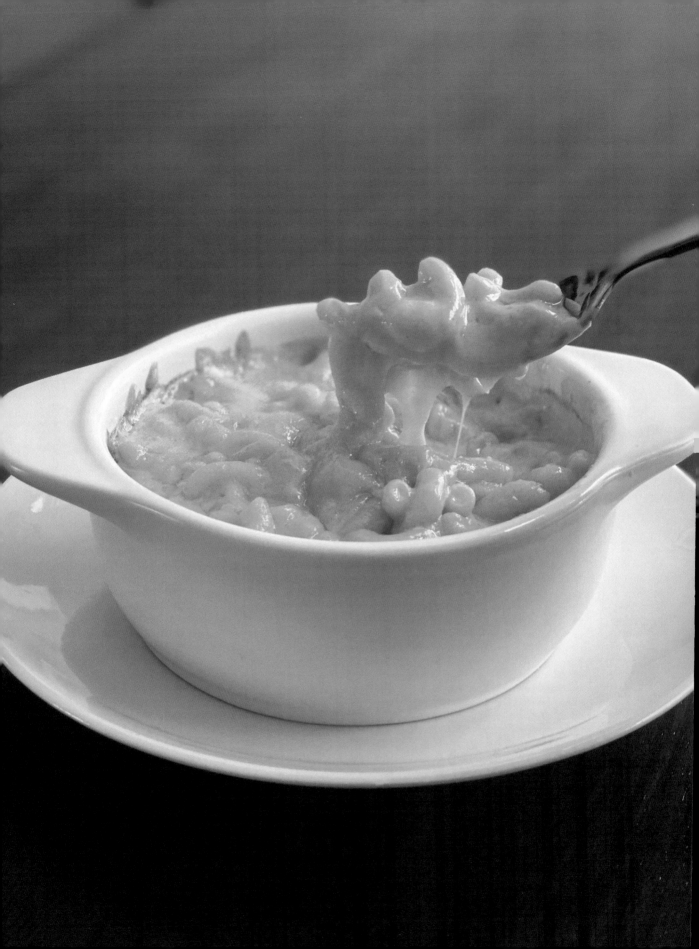

CREAMY MACARONI & CHEESE

Ingredients

1 8-ounce package low-carb pasta*

3 cups sharp cheddar cheese (reserve 1 cup for topping)

½ cup sour cream

4 tablespoons butter

1 cup heavy whipping cream

2 eggs

1 teaspoon salt

½ teaspoon white pepper

½ teaspoon dry mustard powder

Directions

1. Preheat oven to 375°F and grease a 9x13 baking dish.
2. In a large pot, boil pasta according to the directions, drain water, and return pasta to the pot.
3. Stir in butter with the warm pasta. Sprinkle in 2 cups of sharp cheddar cheese and mix well until melted.
4. In a small mixing bowl, whisk together sour cream, eggs, heavy cream, salt, pepper, and mustard and set aside.
5. With your 9x13 baking dish, add half of the pasta, top with ½ cup of cheese, and the add the remaining pasta. Pour the cream mixture over the pasta and top with the remaining cheese.
6. Cover loosely with foil and bake for 20 minutes.
7. Remove foil and turn oven to broil. Continue to cook for an additional 5 minutes to get a crispy cheesy top.

EAT ME

*Find pasta options on page xvi.

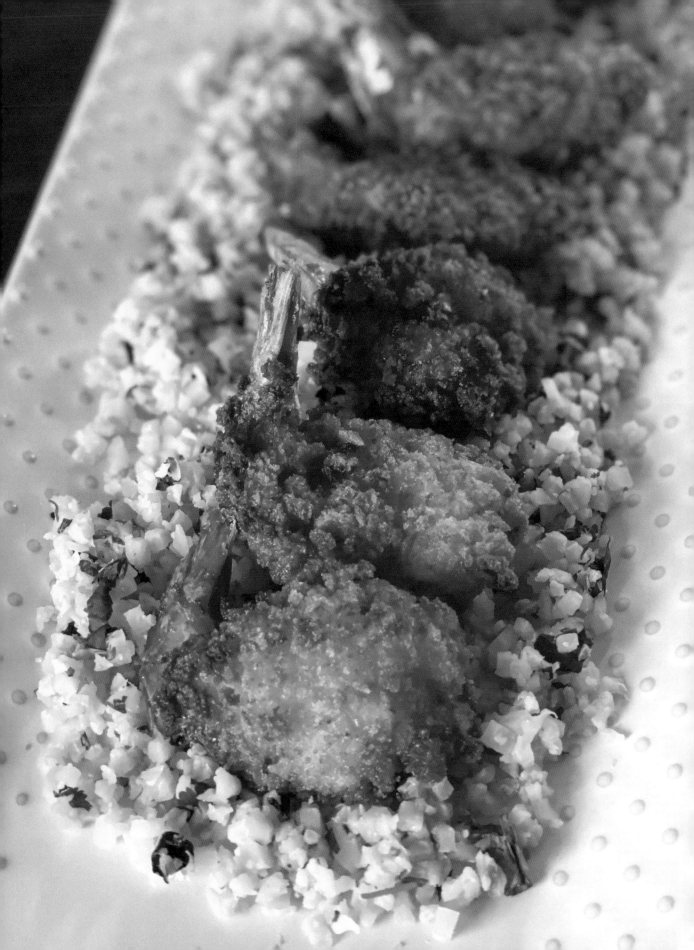

Prep Time: 10 minutes
Cook Time: 15 minutes
Yield: 4 servings

COCONUT SHRIMP WITH CILANTRO-LIME CAULI-RICE

Ingredients

COCONUT SHRIMP

1 pound uncooked shrimp, peeled and deveined
1 cup coconut flour
2 eggs, beaten
½ cup pork rind crumbs
1 teaspoon garlic powder
1 teaspoon onion powder
½ cup unsweetened shredded coconut flakes
1 teaspoon salt
½ teaspoon pepper
Splash of cream
2 tablespoons avocado oil

CILANTRO-LIME CAULI-RICE

10-ounce bag frozen riced cauliflower, microwaved
1 ½ teaspoon salt
½ white pepper
Zest of 1 lime
Juice of 1 lime
3 tablespoons cilantro, chopped

Directions

1. Set up a dredging station of 3 bowls. In the first bowl, mix together coconut flour, salt, and pepper. In the next bowl, whisk eggs and add a splash of cream. Finally, in the last bowl, add crushed pork rinds, onion powder, garlic powder, and unsweetened shredded coconut.
2. Dredge shrimp in order from the first bowl to the third bowl.
3. Heat avocado oil in a large skillet on high heat. Add shrimp to pan and shallow fry until golden and crispy.
4. For the cauli-rice, heat 1 tablespoon avocado oil in a skillet over medium-high heat.
5. Pour in cooked cauliflower and sauté until the moisture is evaporated
6. Stir in salt, pepper, lime zest and juice. Add 3 chopped cilantro, fluff cauli-rice with a fork.

Pro Tip

Shrimp can also be cooked in the air fryer at 400°F for three minutes on each side.

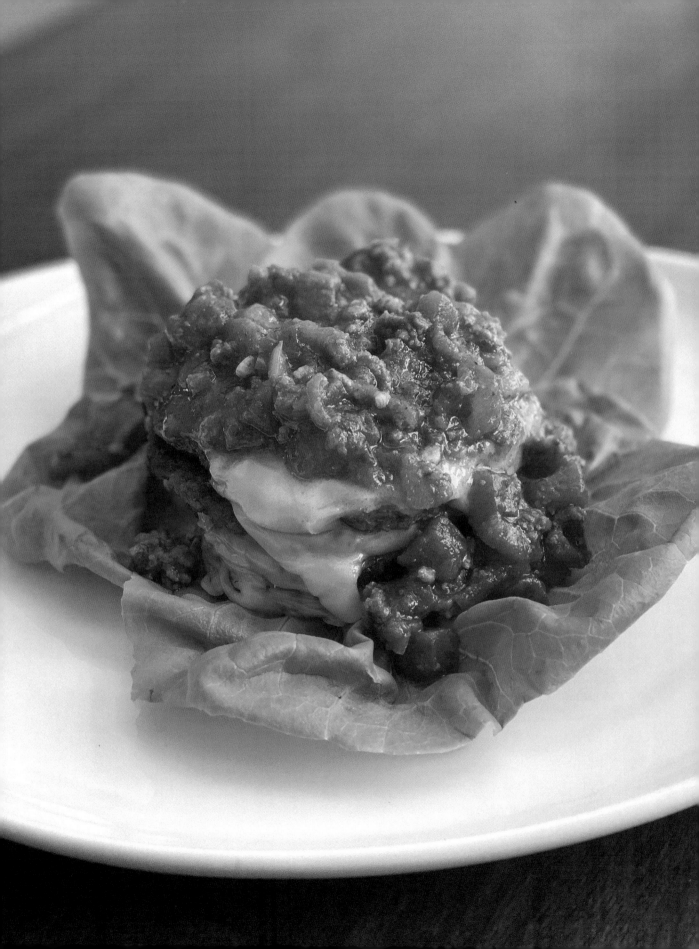

Prep Time: 5 minutes
Cook Time: 10 minutes
Yield: 4 servings

CHILI CHEESEBURGER

Ingredients

1 pound ground beef
Low-carb hamburger bun (optional)
2 cups prepared chili*
4 slices sharp cheddar cheese
Lettuce
Tomato
Red onion
Mayo
Mustard
No-sugar-added ketchup

Directions

1. Season and cook burger to your preference.
2. Top with cheese and melt. Assemble burger with desired toppings and then top with chili.

Pro Tip

Serve open-face style on a low-carb bun**.

*Chili recipe on page 75.
**Find hamburger bun options on page xvi.

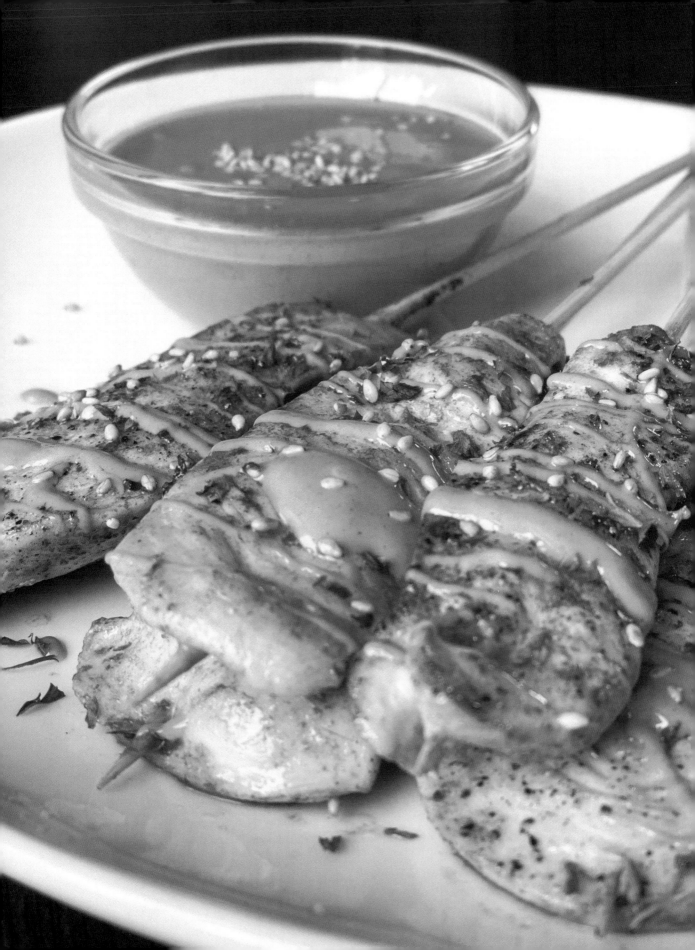

CHICKEN SATAY WITH PEANUT SAUCE

Ingredients

CHICKEN

4 chicken breasts sliced into strips
1 tablespoon lime juice
1 tablespoon rice wine vinegar
2 tablespoons soy sauce or coconut aminos
1 tablespoon avocado oil
1 teaspoon minced garlic
1 teaspoon minced ginger
1 teaspoon chili powder
1 teaspoon granular sweetener

PEANUT SAUCE

½ cup creamy natural peanut butter
1 teaspoon minced ginger
1 teaspoon minced garlic
1 tablespoon chopped jalapeño
2 tablespoons rice wine vinegar
1 tablespoon lime juice
2 tablespoons water
2 tablespoons powdered sweetener

Directions

1. Whisk together lime juice, rice wine vinegar, soy sauce, avocado oil, ginger, garlic, chili powder, and sweetener in a small bowl.
2. In a large Ziplock bag, add the chicken and the sauce. Shake and marinate in the refrigerator for 1 hour or up to 24 hours.
3. Using the grill, cook chicken for 6 to 8 minutes per side over medium heat.
4. For the peanut sauce, combine all the ingredients in a blender or food processor and blend until smooth.
5. Garnish chicken with fresh chopped parsley, scallions, and serve with peanut sauce.

EAT ME

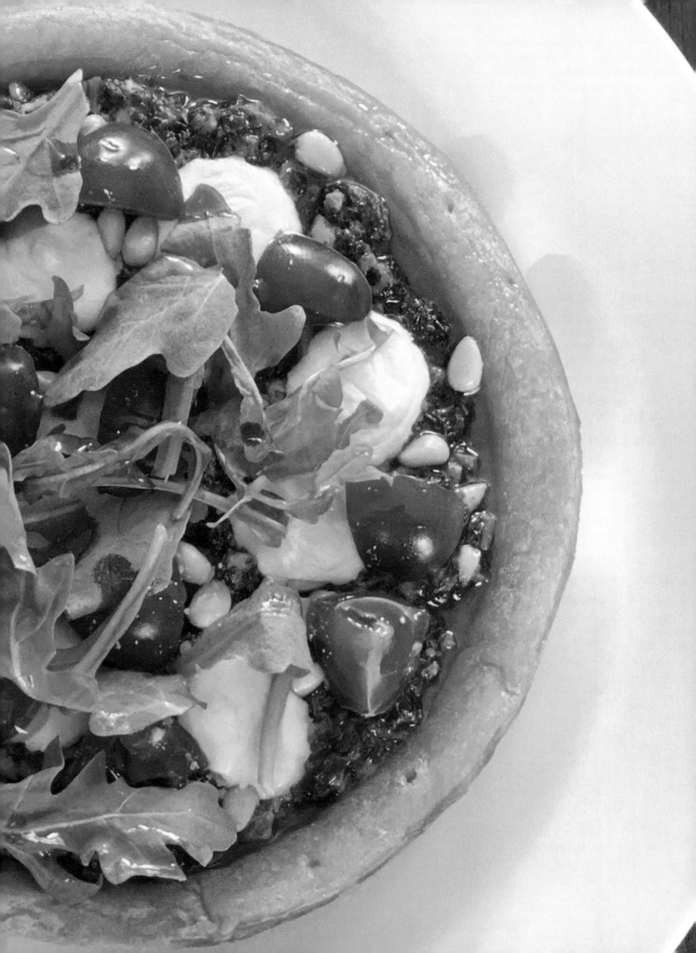

Prep Time: 10 minutes
Cook Time: 20 minutes
Yield: 4 servings

PESTO PIZZA

Ingredients

1 batch prepared fathead dough*
1 batch pesto sauce (recipe below)
1 cup mozzarella cheese, shredded
¼ cup pine nuts
1 handful baby arugula leaves
2 tablespoons olive oil
Heirloom tomatoes (optional)

PESTO SAUCE

2 cups fresh basil leaves
⅓ cup almonds
⅓ cup freshly grated parmesan cheese
2 tablespoons minced garlic
⅓ cup olive oil
Juice of half a lemon
½ teaspoon salt
¼ teaspoon pepper

Directions

1. Preheat oven to 425°F.
2. Place chilled fathead dough between two pieces of parchment paper. Using a rolling pin, roll out dough and then place on a vented pizza pan lined with parchment paper. Pierce the dough with a fork and bake for 10-12 minutes until lightly golden.
3. For the pesto, combine all the ingredients in a blender and pulse until smooth.
4. Spread the pesto onto the crust. Add the mozzarella cheese and pine nuts.
5. Return to the oven and continue cooking for 8 minutes or until the cheese has melted.
6. Top with baby arugula and a light drizzle of olive oil.

*Fathead dough recipe on page 25.

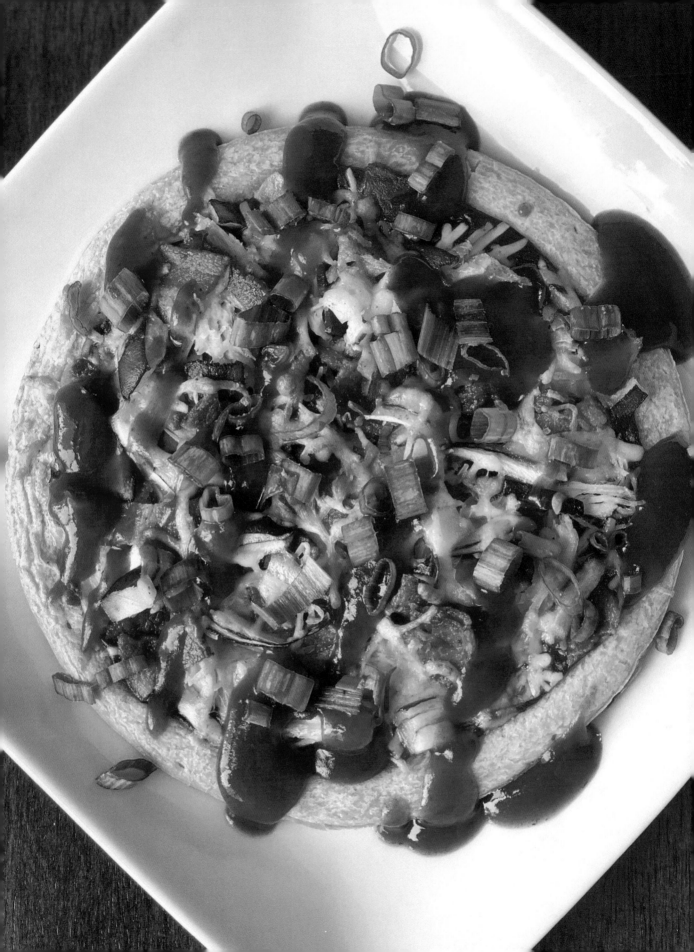

Prep Time: 10 minutes
Cook Time: 20 minutes
Yield: 4 servings

BBQ CHICKEN PIZZA

Ingredients

1 batch prepared fathead dough*
½ cup sugar-free BBQ sauce
6 ounces shredded chicken
3 strips bacon, pan fried and crumbled
¼ cup red onion, chopped
1 cup Colby jack cheese, shredded

Directions

1. Preheat oven to 425°F and line a vented pizza pan with parchment paper.
2. Between two sheets of parchment paper, roll out fathead dough and transfer to the vented pizza pan. Pierce the crust with a fork to prevent air pockets from forming while baking.
3. Bake 10-12 minutes until lightly golden and then remove from oven.
4. Spread BBQ sauce evenly onto the crust. Top with remaining ingredients and return to the oven for an additional 5-8 minutes.

*Fathead dough recipe on page 25.

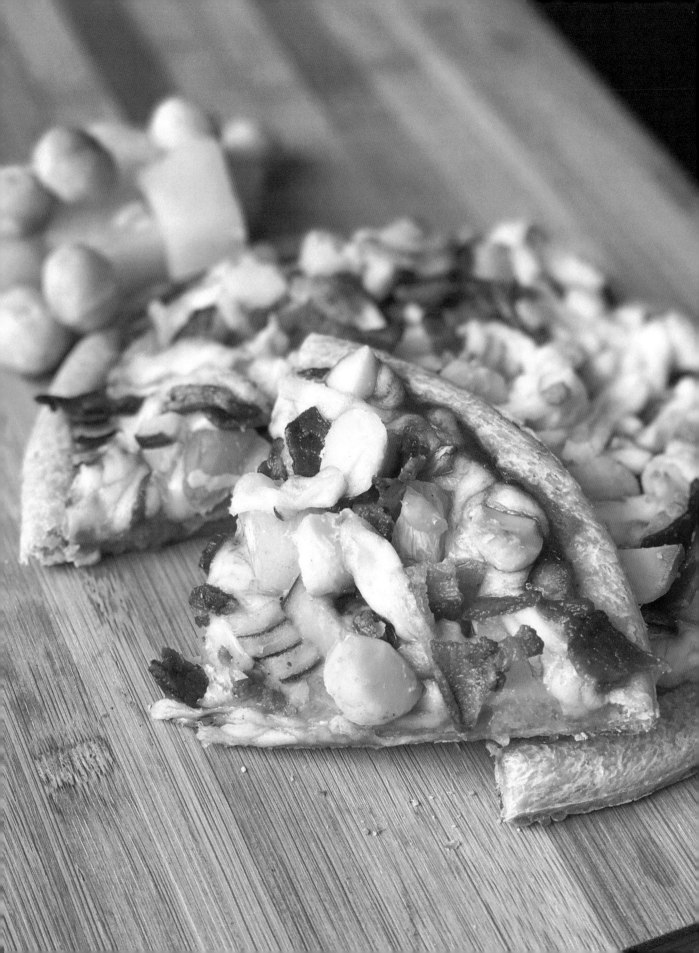

Prep Time: 10 minutes
Cook Time: 20 minutes
Yield: 4 servings

NUTTY HAWAIIAN PIZZA

Ingredients

1 batch prepared fathead dough*
½ cup Rao's no-sugar-added marinara sauce
1 package sliced Canadian bacon
3 strips bacon, pan fried and crumbled
¼ cup pineapple tidbits, drained
¼ cup macadamia nuts, chopped
1 cup mozzarella cheese, shredded

Directions

1. Preheat oven to 425°F and line a vented pizza pan with parchment paper.
2. Between two sheets of parchment paper, roll out fathead dough and transfer to the vented pizza pan. Pierce the crust with a fork to prevent air pockets from forming while baking.
3. Bake 10-12 minutes until lightly golden and then remove from oven.
4. Spread marinara sauce evenly onto the crust. Top with remaining ingredients and return to the oven for an additional 5-8 minutes until cheese is melted.

Pro Tip

Dip a slice in some homemade ranch dressing**!

*Fathead dough recipe on page 25.
**Ranch dressing recipe on page 191.

EAT ME

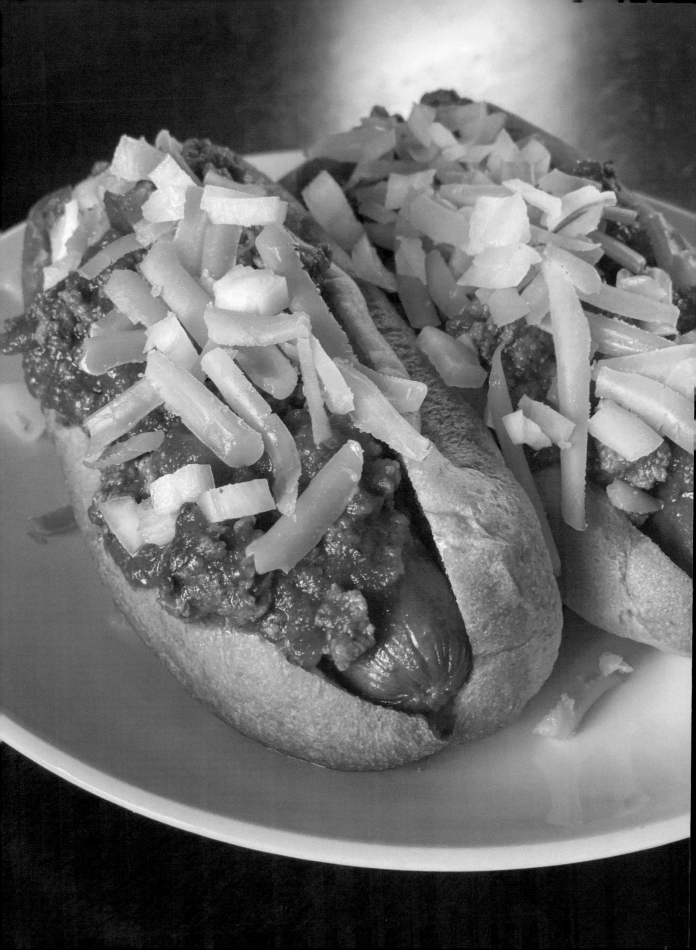

CHILI CHEESE DOG

Ingredients

1 8-count package hotdogs
2 cups prepared chili*
2 cups sharp cheddar cheese, shredded
½ red onion, diced
Low-carb hotdog buns (optional)**

Directions

1. Grill hotdogs or heat in an air fryer.
2. Place cooked hotdogs inside hotdog buns
3. Top with chili, cheese, and onions.

*Chili recipe on page 75.
**Find hotdog bun options on page xvi.

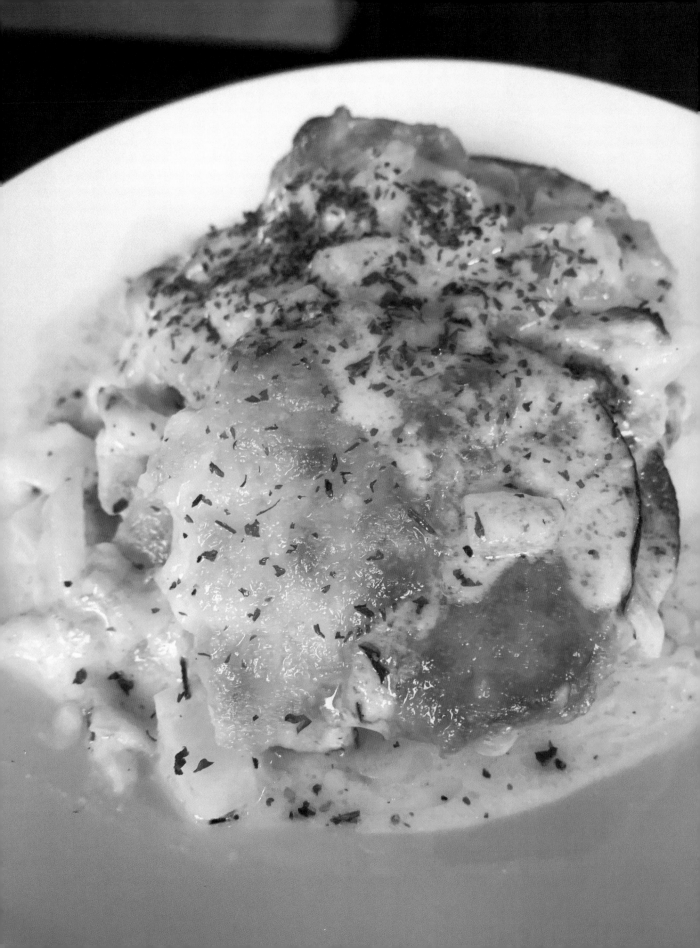

Prep Time: 15 minutes
Cook Time: 25 minutes
Yield: 6 servings

ZUCCHINI AU GRATIN

Ingredients

2 large zucchini or 4 small zucchinis

1 tablespoon butter

½ medium yellow onion, diced

1 cup heavy whipping cream

1 cup parmesan cheese (reserve half for topping)

1 cup mozzarella cheese, shredded (reserve half for topping)

1 teaspoon minced garlic

½ teaspoon salt

½ teaspoon white pepper

1 ½ teaspoons Italian seasoning

1 tablespoon chopped parsley for garnish

Directions

1. Preheat oven to 350°F
2. Slice zucchini in ¼-inch slices and then place on a paper towel to absorb moisture.
3. In a medium saucepan, melt butter over medium-high heat. Sauté onions in butter until soft and translucent. Add minced garlic and cook for 1-2 minutes.
4. Mix in the heavy cream, parmesan cheese, mozzarella cheese, garlic, salt, white pepper, and Italian seasoning. Stir until cheese is melted and sauce has thickened.
5. Grease an 8x8 baking dish with cooking spray.
6. Spread 2 tablespoon of sauce on the bottom of the baking dish and then add in the zucchini. Pour marinara sauce over the zucchini slices and top with the remaining mozzarella and parmesan cheese.
7. Bake for 25 minutes until cheese is golden and bubbly. Garnish with parsley.

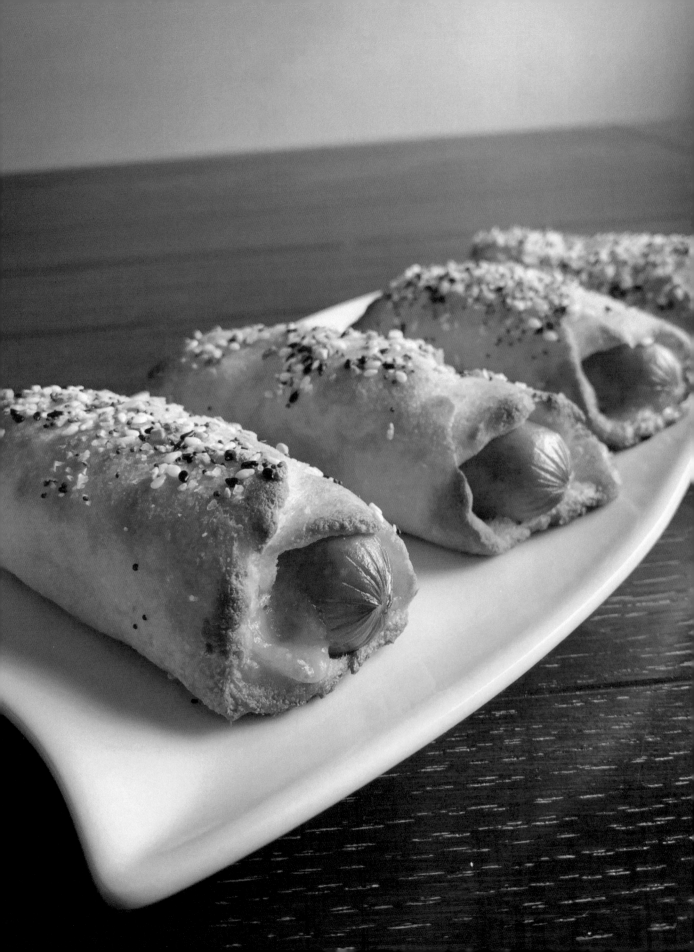

Prep Time: 10 minutes
Cook Time: 18 minutes
Yield: 8 servings

PIGS IN A BLANKET

Ingredients

1 batch prepared fathead dough*
1 8-count package hotdogs
2 cups sharp cheddar cheese, shredded
Everything But the Bagel seasoning (optional)

Directions

1. Preheat oven to 425°F and line a baking sheet with parchment paper.
2. Divide prepared fathead dough into 8 equal parts and roll into balls. Using your hand, flatten each ball and wrap around a hotdog.
3. Place onto baking sheet, seam side down, and sprinkle Everything But the Bagel seasoning over the top.
4. Bake for 15-18 minutes until dough is golden.

*Fathead dough recipe on page 25.

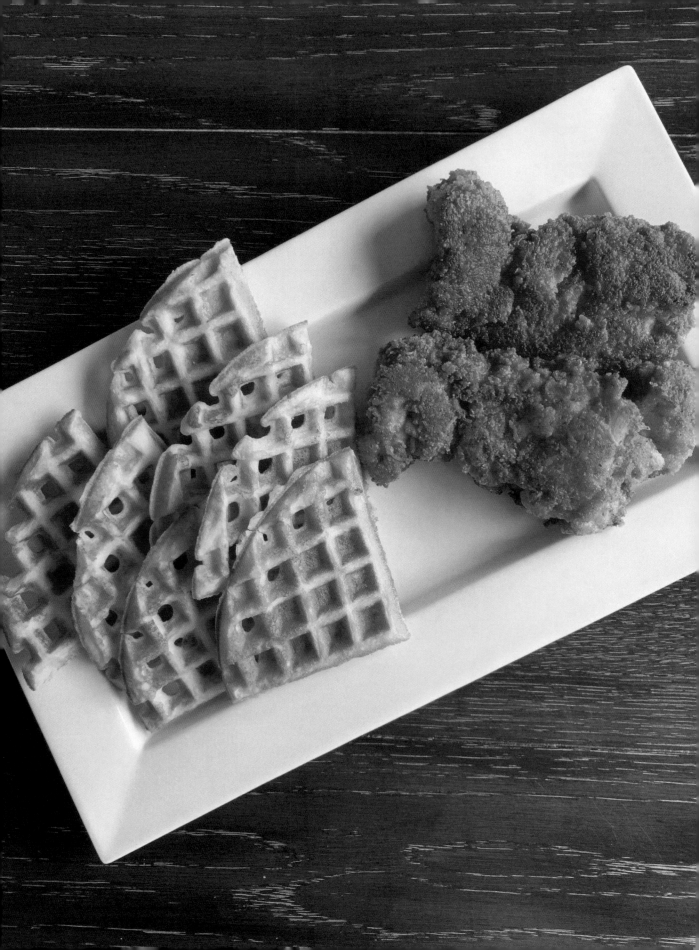

CHICKEN 'N WAFFLES

Ingredients

FRIED CHICKEN

4 boneless, skinless chicken thighs
2 eggs
2 tablespoons heavy whipping cream
¼ cup almond flour
¼ cup parmesan cheese
½ teaspoon paprika
½ teaspoon cayenne pepper
½ teaspoon salt
½ teaspoon pepper
Avocado oil for frying

WAFFLES

1 ¼ cups Carbquik baking mix
1 tablespoon granular sweetener
1 egg, beaten
¼ cup heavy whipping cream
¼ cup unsweetened almond milk
½ teaspoon vanilla extract
2 tablespoons oil

Directions

1. Heat avocado oil in a large frying pan on medium-high heat.
2. In a shallow bowl, beat eggs and whisk in the heavy cream. Using a second shallow bowl, stir together the almond flour, parmesan cheese, paprika, cayenne pepper, salt, and pepper.
3. Pat chicken thighs with a paper towel to remove excess moisture.
4. Coat each thigh in breading first, then the egg wash, and then in the breading again. Shake off the extra breading and place in the hot oil.
5. Shallow fry the chicken thighs until a deep brown color is achieved, approximately 5 minutes on each side.
6. Remove from heat and drain on paper towels.
7. For the waffles, preheat a waffle iron.
8. In a medium mixing bowl, combine Carbquik and granular sweetener.
9. In a separate bowl, beat egg and heavy cream together using an electric hand mixer. Add in almond milk.
10. Pour the wet mixture into the dry ingredient bowl. Stir together, careful not to overmix.
11. Pour batter into waffle iron and cook.

EAT ME

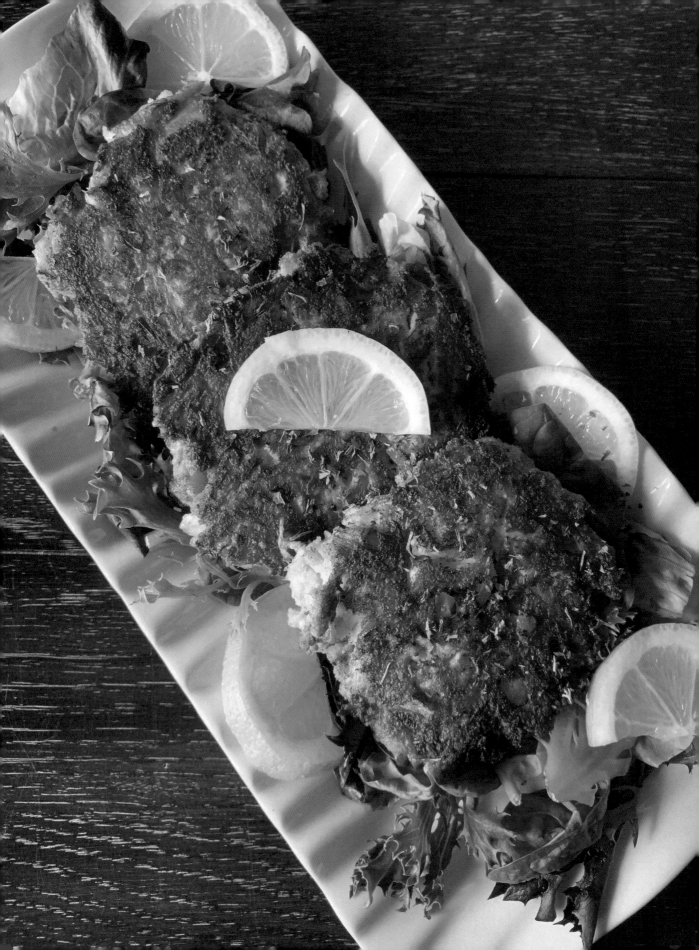

Prep Time: 5 minutes
Cook Time: 10 minutes
Yield: 4 servings

CRAB CAKES

Ingredients

16 ounces lump crab meat
½ red bell pepper, finely diced
½ yellow onion, finely diced
¼ cup mayonnaise
½ cup almond flour
1 tablespoon Old Bay seasoning
2 eggs, slightly beaten
Cracked pepper to taste
Butter for frying

Directions

1. In a large mixing bowl, add all ingredients and mix well.
2. Form into patties and chill in the freezer for 10 minutes.
3. In a large frying pan, melt some butter. Fry crab cakes in butter until golden. Flip, and continue to fry. Crab cakes will be delicate, so handle with care while cooking.
4. Drain on a paper towel and enjoy!

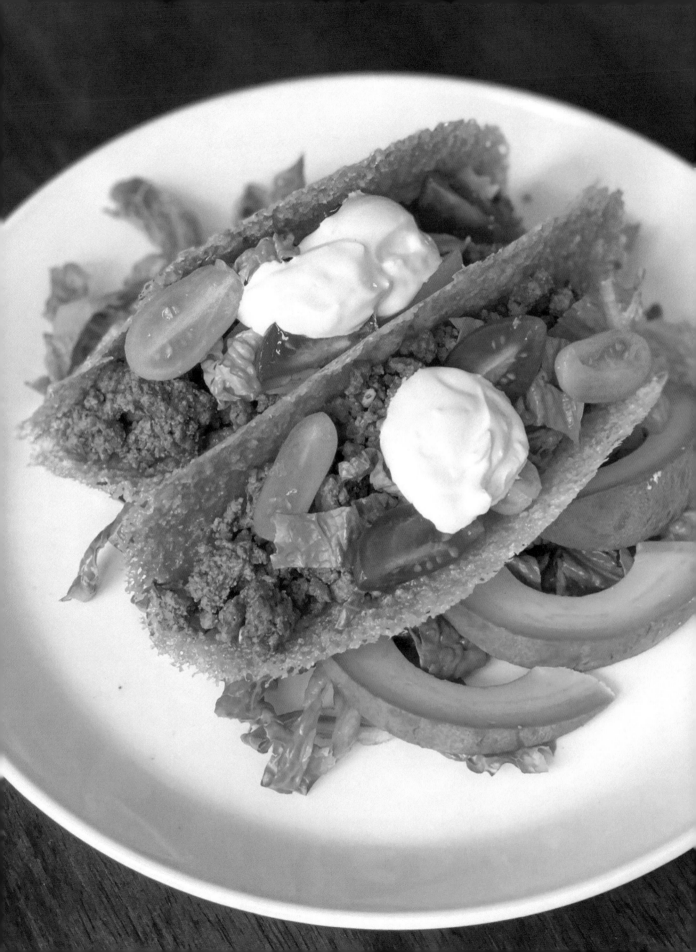

CRISPY CHEESE SHELL TACOS

Ingredients

1 pound ground beef
½ cup diced white onion
1 tablespoon minced garlic
1 teaspoon salt
½ teaspoon pepper
3 tablespoons taco seasoning*
2 cups shredded cheese

Directions

1. Brown hamburger meat in a medium skillet and drain.
2. Add onion and garlic and cook for five minutes.
3. Stir in taco seasoning and mix well.
4. To make the cheese shells, place 1/3 cup of shredded on parchment paper and form into a 4-inch round. Microwave for 90 seconds.
5. Using the parchment paper fold the cheese over to form a shell and place it between two objects to allow it to cool and crisp up.
6. Fill shells with taco meat and toppings of your choice: Lettuce, diced tomatoes, sour cream, onions, queso blanco**, hot sauce, extra cheese, or fresh cilantro.

*Taco Seasoning recipe on page 181.
**Queso blanco recipe on page 33.

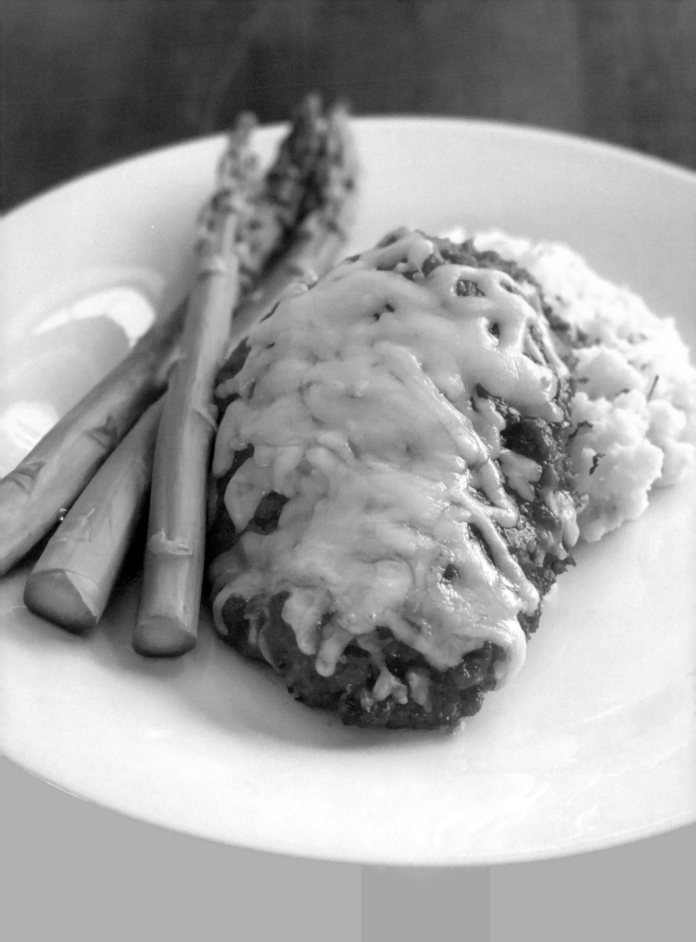

Prep Time: 5 minutes
Cook Time: 25 minutes
Yield: 4 servings

CHICKEN PARMESAN

Ingredients

1 pound boneless, skinless chicken breast
⅓ cup almond flour
⅓ cup parmesan cheese
1 teaspoon garlic powder
½ teaspoon salt
2 cups Rao's no-sugar-added marinara sauce
2 cups mozzarella cheese, shredded
Avocado oil for frying

Directions

1. Preheat oven to 375°F.
2. Trim chicken and use a meat mallet to pound chicken into ½-inch fillets.
3. On a plate, mix together the almond flour, parmesan cheese, garlic powder, and salt.
4. In a large frying pan, heat avocado oil over medium heat.
5. Dip chicken breast into almond flour mixture and coat all sides. Place into the hot skillet and fry until golden, about 5 minutes for each side.
6. Remove from pan and drain on paper towels.
7. In a 9x13 baking dish, spread ¼ cup of marinara sauce over the bottom. Add the fried chicken in a single layer. Pour remaining marinara sauce over the chicken and top with the mozzarella cheese.
8. Bake for 10-15 minutes until cheese is melted.

Pro Tip

Serve over a bed of mashed cauliflower or keto pasta*.

*Keto pasta options on page xvi.

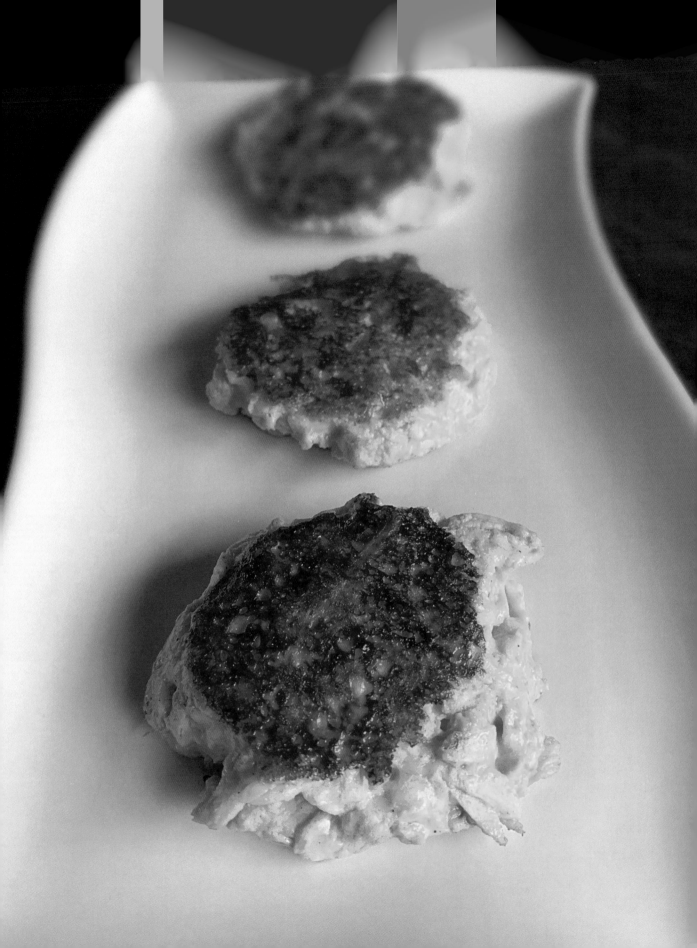

BUFFALO CHICKEN PATTIES

Ingredients

12 ounces shredded chicken
¾ cup mozzarella cheese, shredded
3 ounces cream cheese, softened
3 tablespoons buffalo sauce
Butter for frying

Directions

1. In a large mixing bowl, combine all ingredients until incorporated.
2. Form mixture into patties and chill in the freezer for 10 minutes.
3. In a large frying pan, melt the butter on medium-high heat.
4. Remove chicken patties from freezer and fry until a golden cheese crust forms. Flip, and continue to fry on other side. Patties are delicate, so handle with care while frying.

WHIPPED &

Apple Cobbler

Chocolate Chip Pecan
Pie Bars

Churro Truffles

Butter Rum Cake

Coconut Macaroons

Chocolate Cupcakes with
Chocolate Buttercream

Apple Pie Pizza

Crema de Limón Bark

Chocolate Chip Cookies

No-Bake Quickie Peanut
Butter Bars

Grasshopper Milkshake

Fudgy as F*ck Ganache
Brownies

Pumpkin Mousse with
Spiced Whipped Cream

Vanilla Bean Ice Cream
with Buttery Bourbon
Sauce

Peanut Butter Blondies

Sweet & Spicy Midnight
Bark

CREAMED

Vanilla Rum Bread Pudding

Apple Turn-(Me)-Over

Chocolate Peanut Butter Ice Cream

Cheesecake Bites

Peanut Butter Pie

Tuxedo Shortbread Cookies

White Chocolate Peanut Butter Bark

French Silk Pie

Chocolate Orange Mug Cake

Maple Pecan Spice Mug Cake

Chocolate Peanut Butter Mug Cake

Lemon Poppy Seed Mug Cake

Cocoa Bunny Mug Cake

Russian Tea Cakes

Drunken Pumpkin Cheesecake

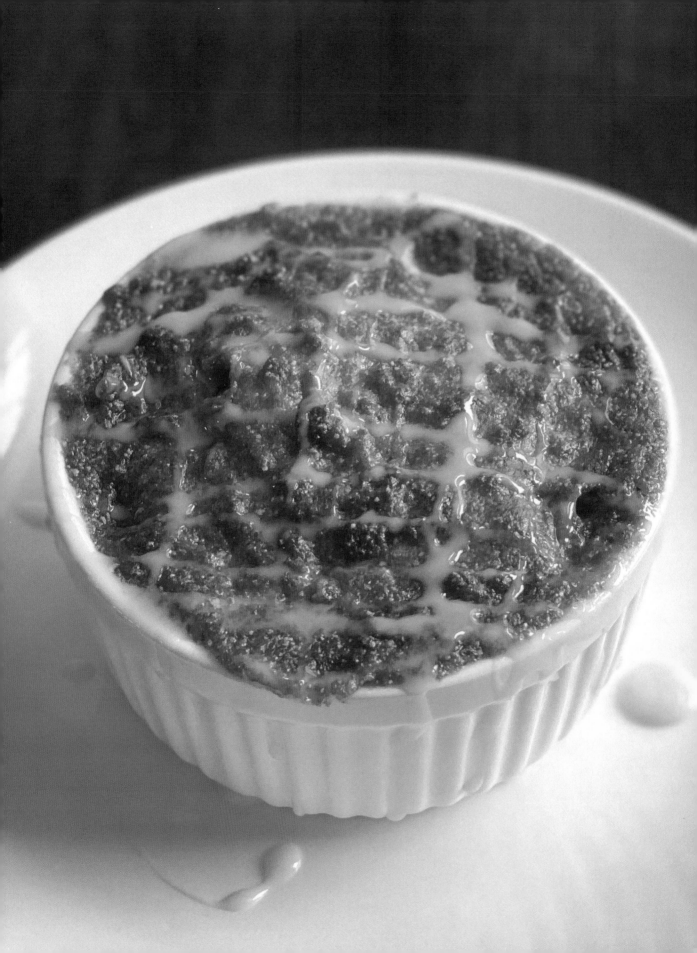

Prep Time: 40 minutes
Cook Time: 25 minutes
Yield: 12 servings

APPLE COBBLER

Ingredients

Directions

4 chayotes

2 tablespoons butter

3 tablespoons Swerve brown sugar replacement

3 tablespoons sugar-free pancake syrup

1 teaspoon ground cinnamon

1 ½ teaspoons pumpkin pie spice

½ teaspoon xanthan gum

2 low-carb wraps*

CRUMBLE TOPPING

½ cup almond flour

½ cup pecans, chopped

½ cup almonds, chopped

½ cup granular sweetener

4 tablespoons cold butter, cubed

1. Preheat over to 350°F and grease a 9x13 baking dish.
2. Prep the chayotes by boiling them whole, with the skin on, for 25-30 mins until fork tender. Set aside to cool.
3. Using a vegetable peeler, peel the skin. Slice length-wise and remove the seed with a spoon. Chop into small cubes and place in a bowl lined with paper towels to remove excess moisture while you make the apple pie sauce.
4. Melt butter in a medium-sized pot. Stir in the brown sugar replacement until dissolved.
5. Add the chayote's and mix to combine.
6. Mix in the rest of ingredients, except the xanthan gum, and stir to combine.
7. Simmer for a few minutes while occasionally stirring.
8. At this time, if you want the sauce thicker, add the xanthan gum and stir.
9. Remove from heat and allow the sauce to continue to thicken as it cools.
10. For the crumble topping, add the almond flour, chopped pecans and almonds, cinnamon, salt, monk fruit, and cold butter to a mixing bowl. Mix with your hands until ingredients are moist and crumbly.
11. Add topping to the cobbler and bake for 20-25 minutes or until golden and bubbly.

Pro Tip

Serve with a scoop of vanilla bean ice cream**.

*Find wrap options on page xvi.

**Vanilla bean ice cream recipe on page 143.

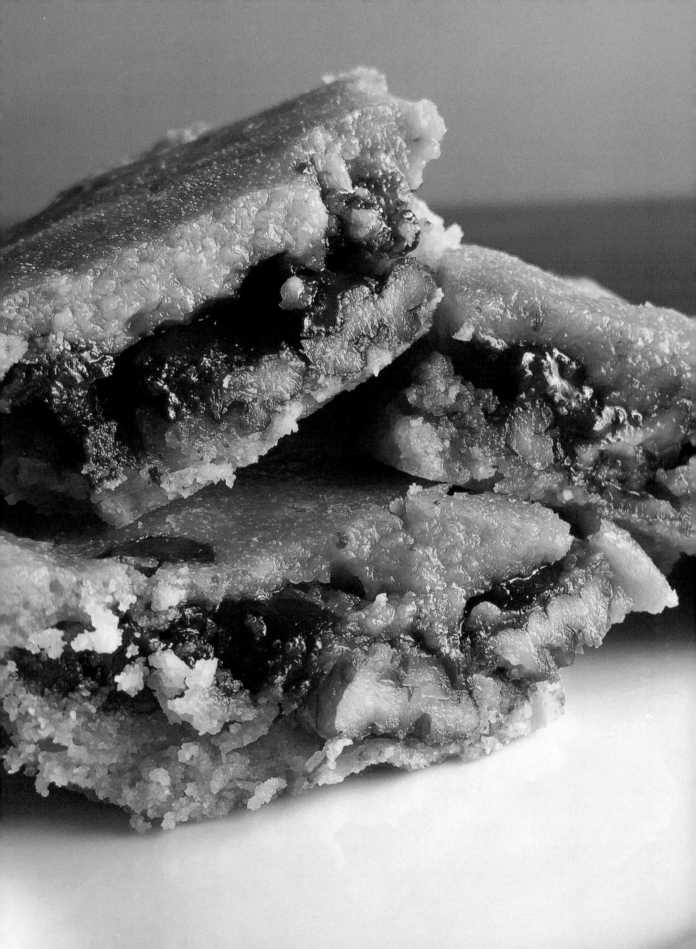

CHOCOLATE CHIP PECAN PIE BARS

Ingredients

CRUST

1 ¼ cups almond flour

¼ cup granular sweetener

⅛ teaspoon salt

¼ cup cold butter, cut into small cubes

PECAN PIE FILLING

½ cup butter

⅔ cup powdered sweetener

1 teaspoon sugar-free pancake syrup

1 ½ teaspoons vanilla extract

½ cup heavy whipping cream

2 eggs

¼ teaspoon salt

1 cup pecan halves, lightly toasted

¼ cup no-sugar-added chocolate chips

Directions

1. Preheat oven to 325°F.
2. Using a food processor, mix the almond flour, granular sweetener, and salt. Add butter and pulse until crumbly.
3. Press crust mixture into the bottom of an 8x8 baking dish.
4. Bake for 10-12 minutes until the edges start to golden.
5. For the filling, melt the butter in a medium saucepan over low heat. Whisk in the powdered sweetener and pancake syrup until combined and then remove from heat.
6. Stir in the vanilla extract and heavy whipping cream before whisking in the eggs and salt.
7. Sprinkle the pecans and chocolate chips over the crust and then pour in the filling.
8. Bake 20-25 minutes until the filling is mostly set. Remove from oven and allow to cool for a minimum of 30 minutes before cutting into them.

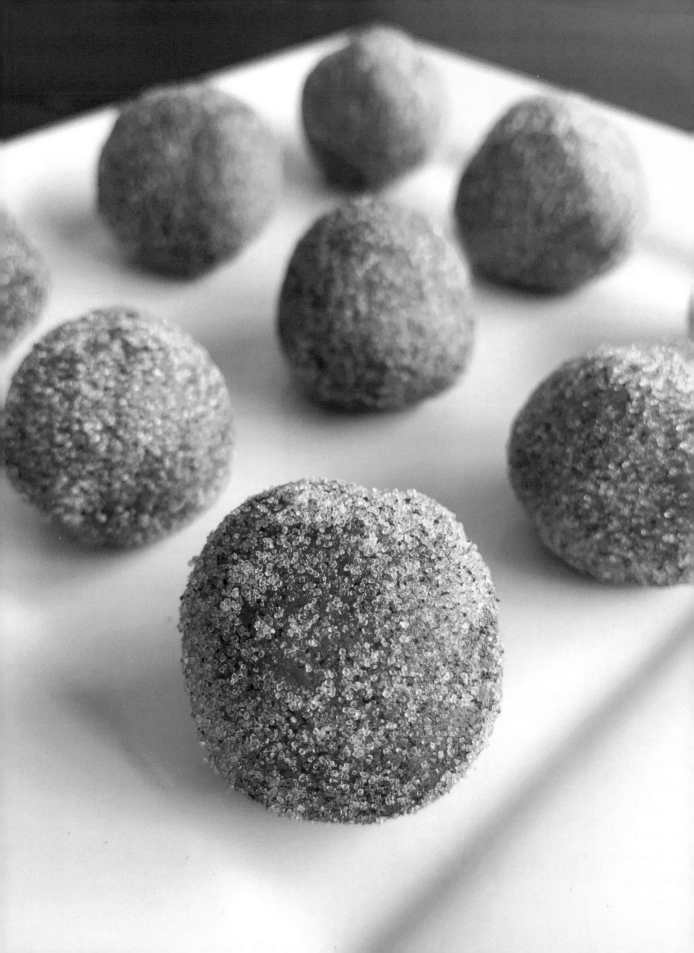

Prep Time: 8 minutes
Cook Time: 0 minutes
Yield: 12 servings

CHURRO TRUFFLES

Ingredients

Directions

TRUFFLES

1 cup almond flour
¼ cup powdered sweetener
½ teaspoon cream of tartar
½ teaspoon ground cinnamon
Pinch of salt
2 tablespoons butter, melted
1 ounce cream cheese, softened
½ teaspoon vanilla extract

COATING

2 tablespoons granular sweetener
1 teaspoon ground cinnamon

1. In a medium mixing bowl, whisk together the almond flour, granular sweetener, cream of tartar, cinnamon, and salt. Add melted butter, softened cream cheese, and vanilla. Mix until well combined.
2. Form the dough into 1-inch balls, squeezing dough together as you do.
3. In a shallow bowl, stir together granular sweetener and cinnamon. Roll truffles in the mixture until coated.

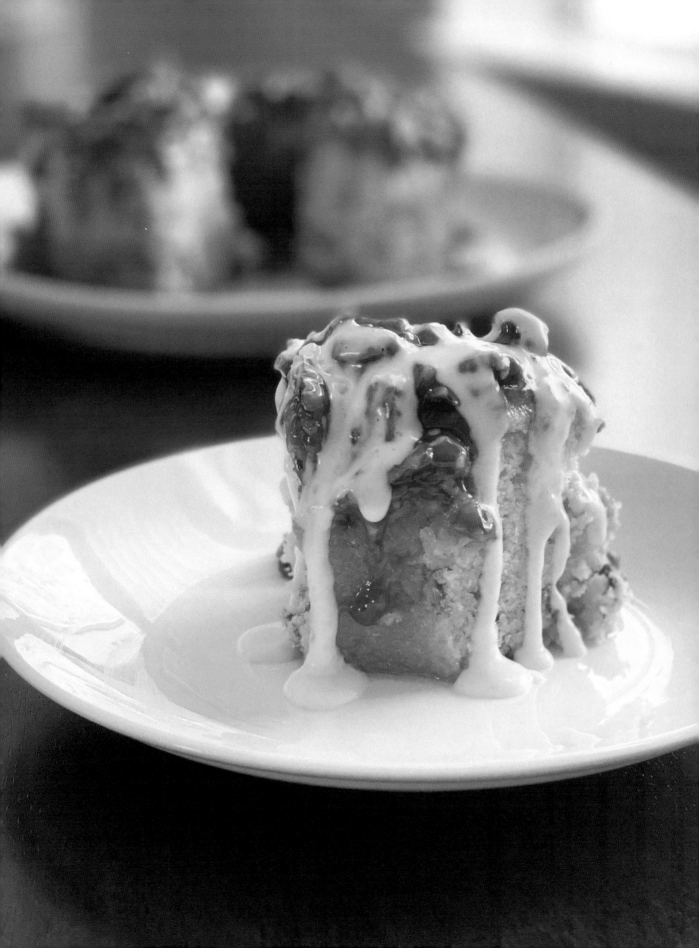

Prep Time: 20 minutes
Cook Time: 35 minutes
Yield: 8 servings

BUTTER RUM CAKE

Ingredients

Directions

CAKE

2 ½ cups almond flour

3 teaspoons baking powder

1 cup powdered sweetener

1 teaspoon vanilla extract

¼ cup butter, melted

¼ cup sour cream

½ cup dark rum

1 teaspoon rum extract

3 eggs at room temperature

WALNUT TOPPING

¾ cup walnuts, chopped

½ cup butter, melted

3 tablespoons powdered sweetener

GLAZE

¼ cup butter, melted

3 tablespoons powdered sweetener

1 teaspoon vanilla extract

2 tablespoons dark rum

2 tablespoons heavy whipping cream

1. Preheat the oven to 350°F.
2. To make the topping, add 2 tablespoons of butter to a medium saucepan and melt on medium-low heat. Add powdered sweetener and chopped walnuts. Mix well and allow to cook for a few minutes until the walnuts are fragrant. Turn the heat off and set to the side while you make the cake batter.
3. In a large mixing bowl, cream the butter and powdered sweetener with an electric hand mixer until combined. Beat in the sour cream, vanilla extract, dark rum, rum extract, and eggs.
4. Gently stir in the almond flour and baking powder until the ingredients are incorporated. Do not over mix.
5. Grease a Bundt cake pan. Pour the cooled walnut cake topping into the bottom of the Bundt pan and spread in an even layer.
6. Next, pour in the cake batter and bake for 35 minutes or until a toothpick comes out clean.
7. To make the glaze, heat the butter, powdered sweetener, vanilla extract, and dark rum in a medium saucepan over medium heat for 8-10 minutes while stirring frequently.
8. Once the glaze has thickened, remove from heat and stir in the heavy whipping cream. Glaze will continue to thicken as it cools
9. When the sides of the cake start to pull away from the pan, carefully invert your Bundt pan onto a cake platter and it should come out with no resistance.
10. Drizzle the warm glaze on top of the cake and serve by itself, with fresh whipped cream, or with sugar-free ice cream.

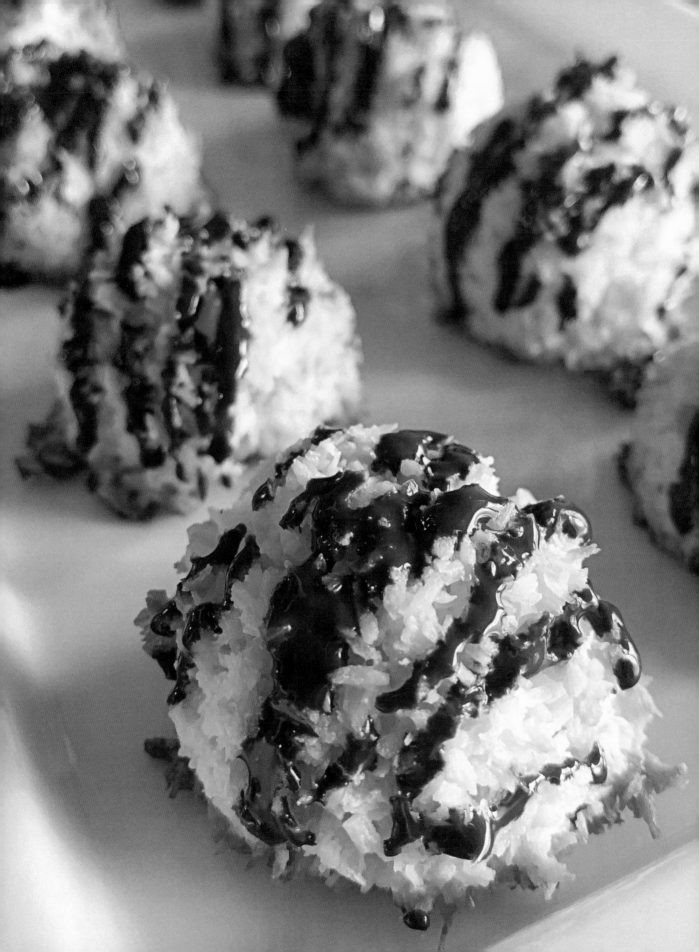

Prep Time: 15 minutes
Cook Time: 20 minutes
Yield: 12 servings

COCONUT MACAROONS

Ingredients

MACAROONS

2 eggs whites, room temperature
1/3 cup granular sweetener
½ teaspoon vanilla extract
½ teaspoon almond extract
¼ teaspoon salt
2 cups unsweetened coconut, shredded

CHOCOLATE DRIZZLE

¼ cup no-sugar-added chocolate chips
½ tablespoon coconut oil

Directions

1. Preheat oven to 325°F and line a baking sheet with parchment paper.
2. Beat egg whites with an electric hand mixer until medium-stiff peaks form. They should move just slightly when you tilt the bowl but not pour out.
3. Slowly add the granular sweetener, 2 tablespoons at a time while beating constantly. Once all the sweetener has been added, beat in the salt, vanilla extract, and almond extract.
4. Using a rubber spatula, gently fold in the coconut flakes, careful to not break down the whites.
5. With a medium cookie scoop, drop the batter onto the parchment paper and bake for 15-20 minutes until lightly golden.
6. While cooling, place chocolate chips and coconut oil in a small microwave-safe bowl and heat in 30-second intervals, stirring in between until chocolate is melted and smooth.
7. Drizzle chocolate over the macaroons and allow to completely cool. Refrigerate for 30 minutes to set the chocolate.

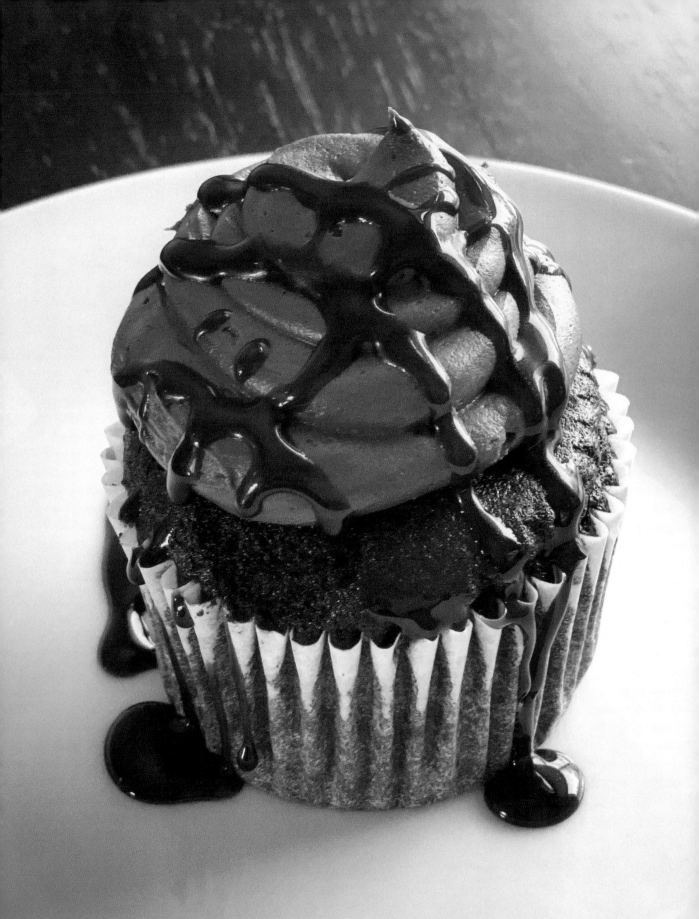

Prep Time: 15 minutes
Cook Time: 20 minutes
Yield: 12 servings

CHOCOLATE CUPCAKES WITH CHOCOLATE BUTTERCREAM

Ingredients

CUPCAKES

1 ½ cups almond flour
½ cup unsweetened cocoa powder
2 teaspoons baking powder
2 tablespoons instant espresso powder
¼ teaspoon salt
½ cup butter, melted
3 eggs at room temperature
½ cup sour cream

BUTTERCREAM FROSTING

8 tablespoons butter, softened
8 ounces cream cheese, softened
½ cup powdered sweetener
1 teaspoon vanilla extract
½ cup heavy whipping cream
2 tablespoons instant espresso, brewed
3 tablespoons unsweetened cocoa powder

Directions

1. Preheat oven to 350°F and line a 12-count muffin tin with cupcake liners.
2. In a large mixing bowl, whisk together the almond flour, cocoa powder, baking powder, espresso powder, and salt.
3. Add in the melted butter, eggs, and sour cream and mix well.
4. Fill the cupcake cavities ¾ of the way with the batter and bake for 18-20 minutes or until a toothpick comes out clean.
5. For the frosting, us an electric hand mixer to beat together the butter and cream cheese until fluffy.
6. In a separate bowl whip together heavy cream, powdered sweetener, vanilla, espresso, and coco powder.
7. Fold together both mixtures until well combined.
8. Allow cupcakes to cool before frosting.

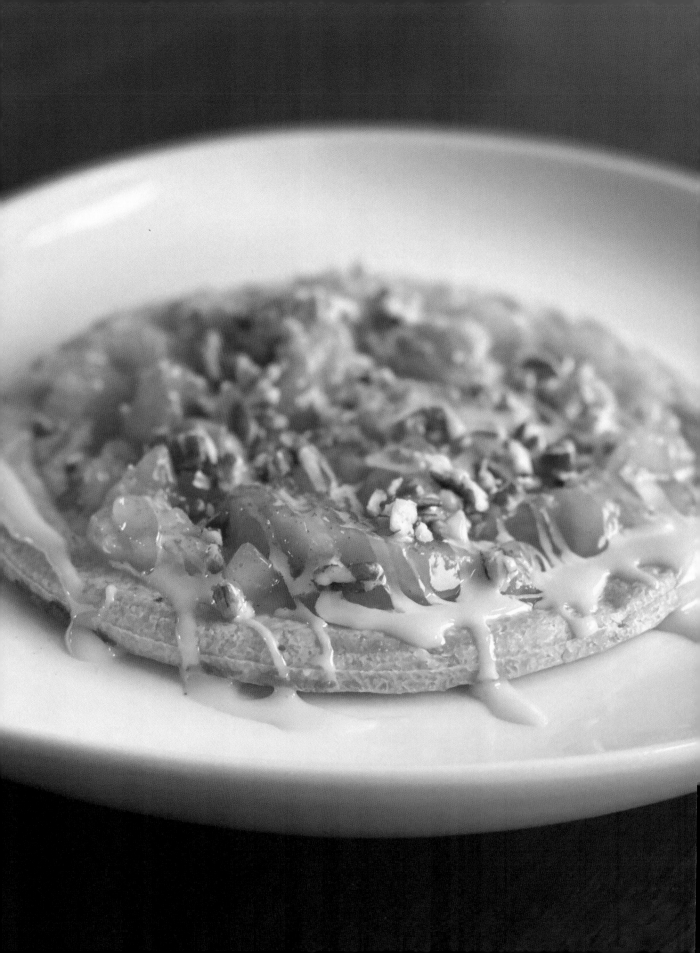

APPLE PIE PIZZA

Ingredients

Directions

PIZZA CRUST

1 batch prepared fathead dough*

APPLE PIE TOPPING

4 chayotes

2 tablespoons butter

3 tablespoons Swerve brown sugar replacement

3 tablespoons sugar-free pancake syrup

1 teaspoon ground cinnamon

1 ½ teaspoons pumpkin pie spice

½ teaspoon xanthan gum (optional)

GLAZE

3 tablespoons heavy whipping cream

2 tablespoons powdered sweetener

1 teaspoon vanilla extract

Pro Tip

Use 10-15 drops of apple pie flavoring from One on One Flavors.

*Fathead dough recipe on page 25.

1. Preheat oven to 425°F.
2. Place chilled fathead dough between two pieces of parchment paper. Using a rolling pin, roll out dough and then place on a vented pizza pan lined with parchment paper. Pierce the dough with a fork and bake for 10-12 minutes until lightly golden.
3. For the filling, boil the chayotes in a large pot, whole with the skin on, for 25-30 minutes until fork tender. Set aside to cool.
4. With a vegetable peeler, remove the skin. Slice chayotes in half, length-wise, and use a spoon to remove the seed. Chop into small cubes and place in a bowl lined with paper towels to soak up excess moisture. Set aside while you make the sauce.
5. Melt butter in a medium-sized pot. Once melted, add the Swerve brown sugar. Stir until dissolved.
6. Add the chayotes and mix to combine.
7. Add the rest of ingredients, except the xanthan gum, and stir to coat the chayotes.
8. On low heat, simmer the mixture for a few minutes while stirring occasionally. As it cooks, the mixture will begin to thicken. If your filling is too thin, add ½ teaspoon of xanthan gum and continue to simmer until the consistency thickens.
9. Remove from heat.
10. Spread apple pie mixture evenly over the top of the crust and return to the oven to bake for 3-5 minutes until heated through.
11. For the glaze, whisk together all ingredients is a small mixing bowl until smooth and drizzle over the pizza.

WHIPPED & CREAMED

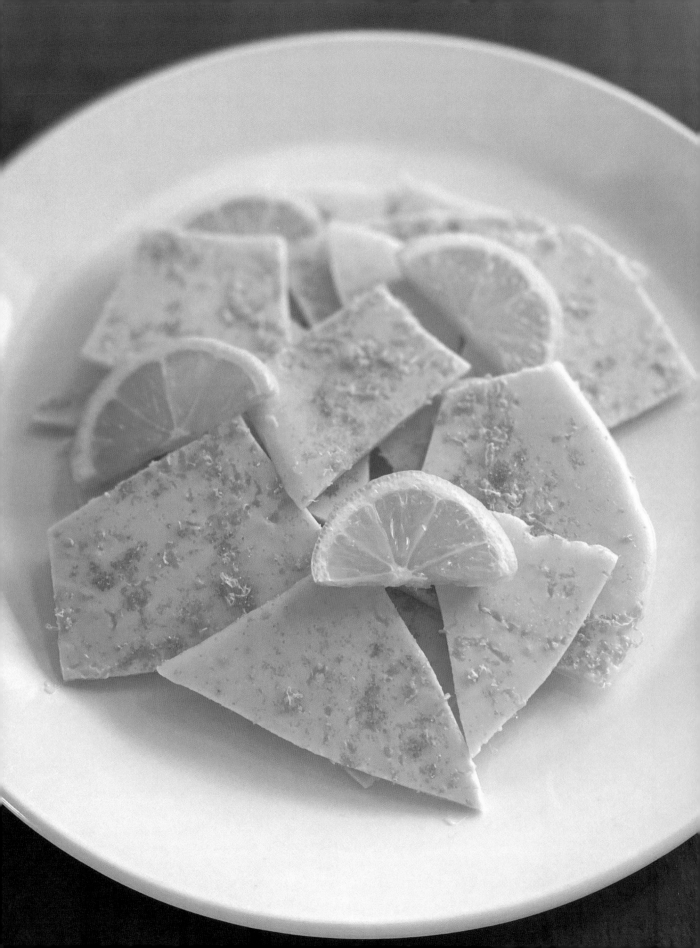

Prep Time: 15 minutes
Cook Time: 0 minutes
Yield: 8 servings

CREMA DE LIMÓN BARK

Ingredients

1 package no-sugar-added white chocolate chips

Zest and juice of 1 whole lemon

½ teaspoon lemon extract

1 teaspoon granular sweetener

Directions

1. Empty the package of white chocolate chips into a microwave-safe bowl and cook in 30-second intervals, stirring in between, until completely melted.
2. Stir in lemon juice, ½ of the zest, and lemon extract.
3. With a rubber spatula, spread mixture onto a baking sheet lined with parchment paper, not to spread too thin.
4. Sprinkle on the remaining lemon zest and granular sweetener. Press gently into the white chocolate to help them stick.
5. Place the baking sheet in the refrigerator for 15-30 minutes or until hardened.
6. Snap bark into pieces and enjoy. Store in an air-tight container in the refrigerator or freezer.

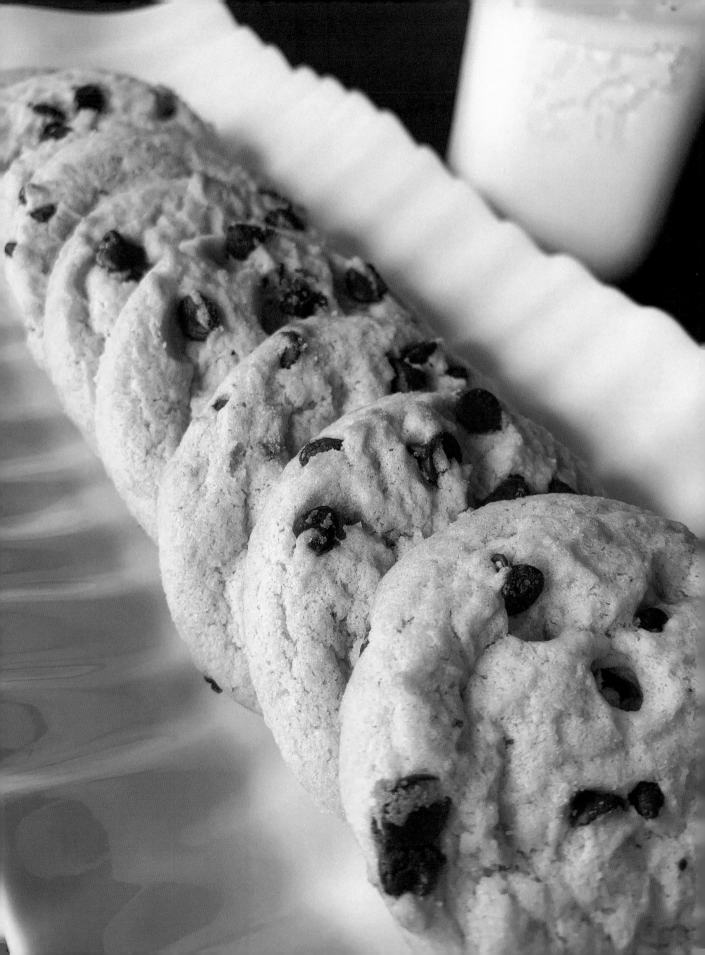

Prep Time: 30 minutes
Cook Time: 10 minutes
Yield: 3 servings

CHOCOLATE CHIP COOKIES

Ingredients

8 tablespoons butter, room temperature
½ cup powdered sweetener
¼ cup Swerve brown sugar replacement
1 egg
1 teaspoon vanilla extract
2 tablespoons heavy whipping cream
1 ⅔ cups almond flour
½ teaspoon baking powder
½ teaspoon xanthan gum
Pinch of salt
⅔ cup no sugar added chocolate chips

Directions

1. Preheat oven to 350°F and line a baking sheet with parchment paper.
2. Using an electric hand mixer, beat together the butter, powdered sweetener, and brown sugar replacement. Mix in the egg, vanilla, and heavy whipping cream.
3. Add in the almond flour, baking powder, xanthan gum, and salt, mixing until well combined.
4. Stir in the chocolate chips.
5. With your hands, roll the dough into 12 balls and place on the baking sheet. Bake for 10 minutes.
6. Remove from oven and let cool for 20 minutes before eating.

Pro Tip

Cookies will be delicate right out of the oven. As they cool, they will become more stable.

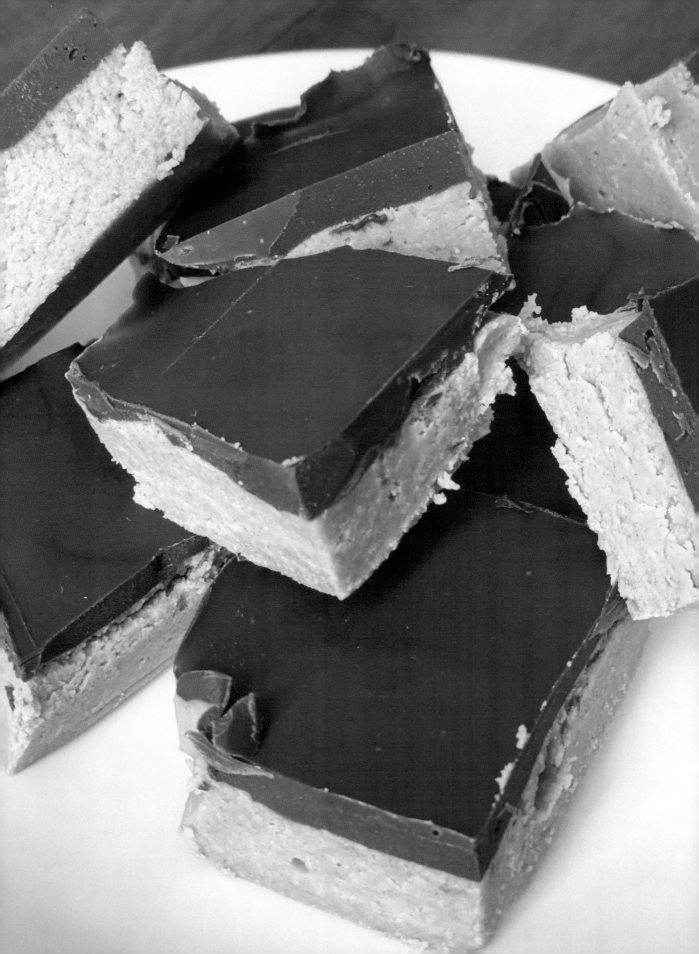

Prep Time: 10 minutes
Cook Time: 0 minutes
Yield: 9 servings

NO-BAKE QUICKIE PEANUT BUTTER BARS

Ingredients

½ cup creamy natural peanut butter
2 tablespoons butter, melted
¾ cup almond flour
1 teaspoon vanilla extract
¾ cup powdered sweetener

CHOCOLATE TOPPING

½ cup no-sugar-added chocolate chips
1 tablespoon butter

Directions

1. In a microwave-safe bowl, heat the peanut butter and butter in 30 second intervals, stirring in between, until melted and smooth.
2. Stir in almond flour, vanilla, and powdered sweetener until combined.
3. Pour mixture into an 8x8 baking dish lined with parchment paper and set aside.
4. For the chocolate topping, combine chocolate chips and butter together in a microwave-safe bowl and heat in 30 second intervals, stirring in between, until melted and smooth.
5. Pour over the top of the peanut butter mixture and transfer to the refrigerator to chill for 30 minutes.
6. Cut into bars and enjoy.

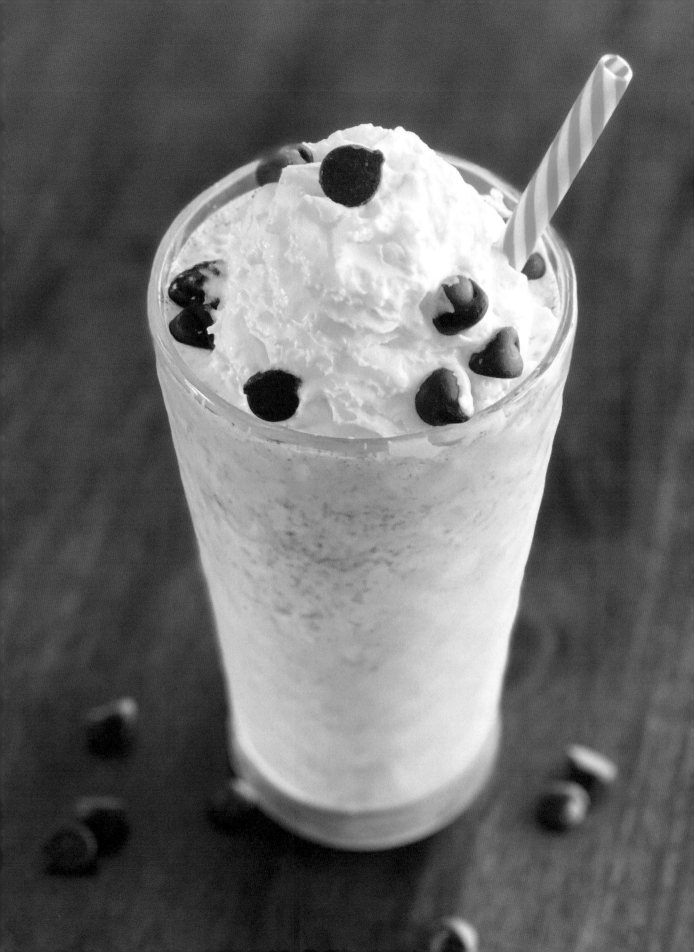

Prep Time: 5 minutes
Cook Time: 0 minutes
Yield: 1 serving

GRASSHOPPER MILK SHAKE

Ingredients

1 cup half & half

4-6 ice cubes

⅛ teaspoon mint extract

2 tablespoons sugar-free chocolate syrup

2 ounces cream cheese, softened

1 drop green food coloring (optional)

Whipped cream for topping

2 tablespoons no-sugar-added chocolate chips for garnish

Directions

1. Place all the ingredients in a blender, except the whipped cream and chocolate chips.
2. Blend until smooth and creamy.
3. Pour in your favorite glass, top with whipped cream and chocolate chips.

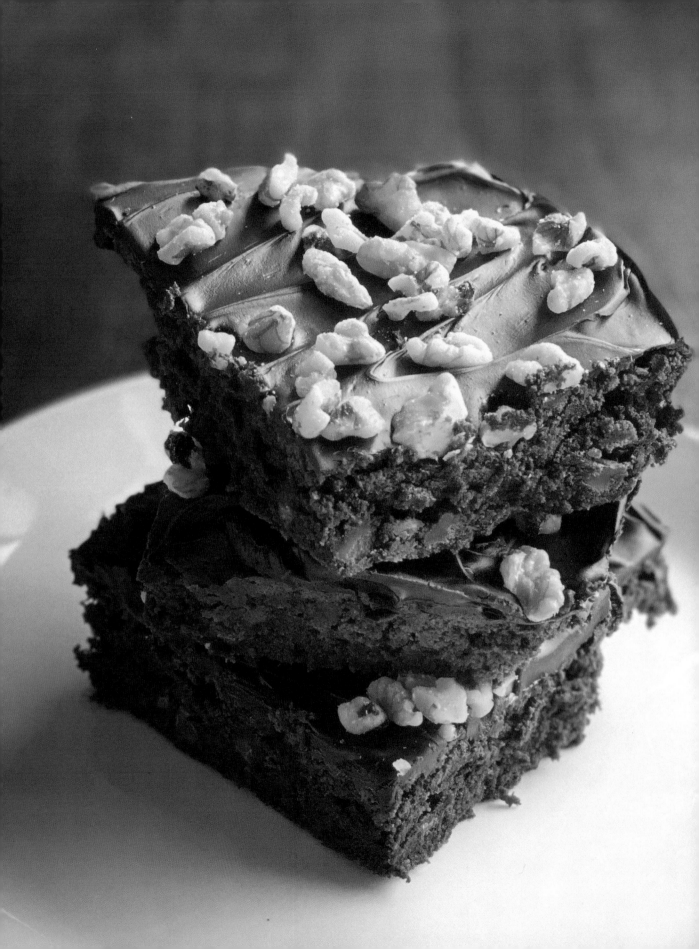

Prep Time: 10 minutes
Cook Time: 18 minutes
Yield: 9 servings

*FUDGY AS F*CK GANACHE BROWNIES*

Ingredients

BROWNIE

½ cup butter

1 cup no-sugar-added chocolate chips (reserve ¼ cup)

¾ cup almond flour

¾ cup powdered sweetener

2 tablespoons unsweetened cocoa powder

1 tablespoon instant espresso powder

2 eggs at room temperature

1 teaspoon vanilla extract

¼ teaspoon salt

CHOCOLATE GANACHE

¾ cup no-sugar-added chocolate chips

½ cup heavy whipping cream

Directions

1. Preheat oven to 350°F. Line an 8x8 baking dish with parchment paper.
2. In a microwave-safe bowl, heat butter and ¾ cup chocolate chips in 30 second intervals, stirring in between until melted.
3. Stir in the flour, powdered sweetener, cocoa powder, espresso powder, eggs, vanilla, and salt to the mixture.
4. Pour the batter into the lined baking dish and sprinkle the remaining ¼ cup of chocolate chips over the top.
5. Bake for 15 -18 minutes or until a toothpick comes out clean.
6. For the ganache, use a double boiler and place the chocolate chips in the bowl to melt. Slowly add heavy cream, stirring constantly, until smooth and glossy.
7. Pour over brownies and enjoy.

Pro Tip

Add chopped nuts, coconut flakes, or peanut butter to the brownie batter.

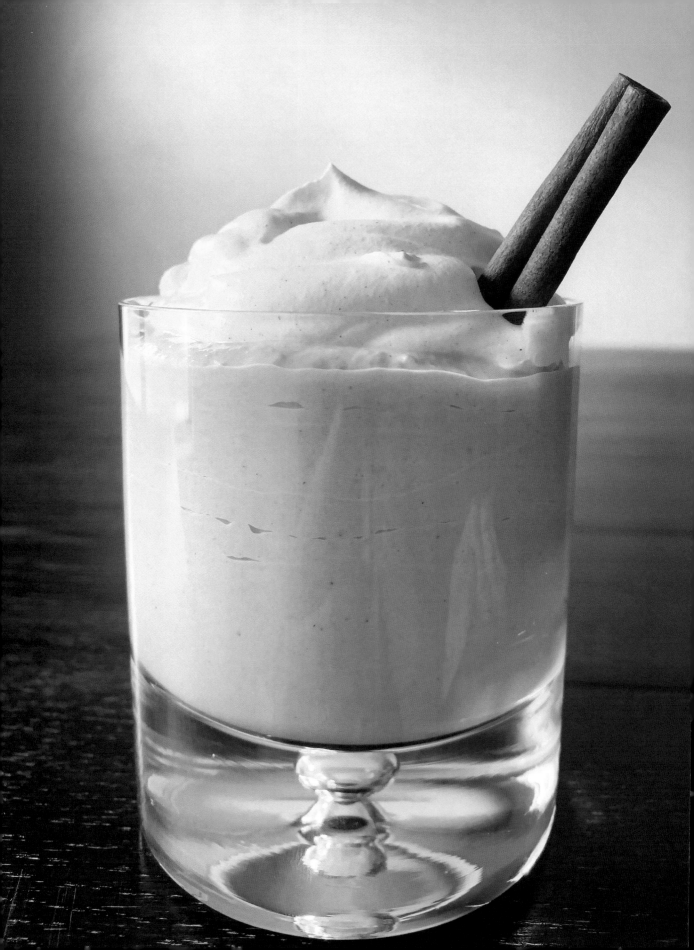

PUMPKIN MOUSSE WITH SPICED WHIPPED CREAM

Ingredients

MOUSSE

1 8-ounce block cream cheese, softened
8 ounces pure pumpkin puree
1 tablespoon pumpkin pie spice
1 teaspoon ground cinnamon
1 teaspoon vanilla extract

SPICED WHIPPED CREAM

1 ½ cups heavy whipping cream
½ teaspoon vanilla extract
1 cup powdered sweetener
1 teaspoon ground cinnamon

Directions

1. For the mousse, use an electric hand mixer to mix the cream cheese, pumpkin puree, pumpkin pie spice, cinnamon, and vanilla until whipped and smooth.
2. Chill in the refrigerator while you prepare the whipped cream.
3. For the whipped cream, pour the heavy whipping cream and vanilla into a large mixing bowl and beat with an electric hand mixer on low while slowly adding the powdered sweetener until stiff peaks form.
4. Add cinnamon and continue to beat.
5. Gently fold in ½ of the whipped cream into the pumpkin mixture.
6. Top with the remaining whipped cream and add a sprinkle of cinnamon.

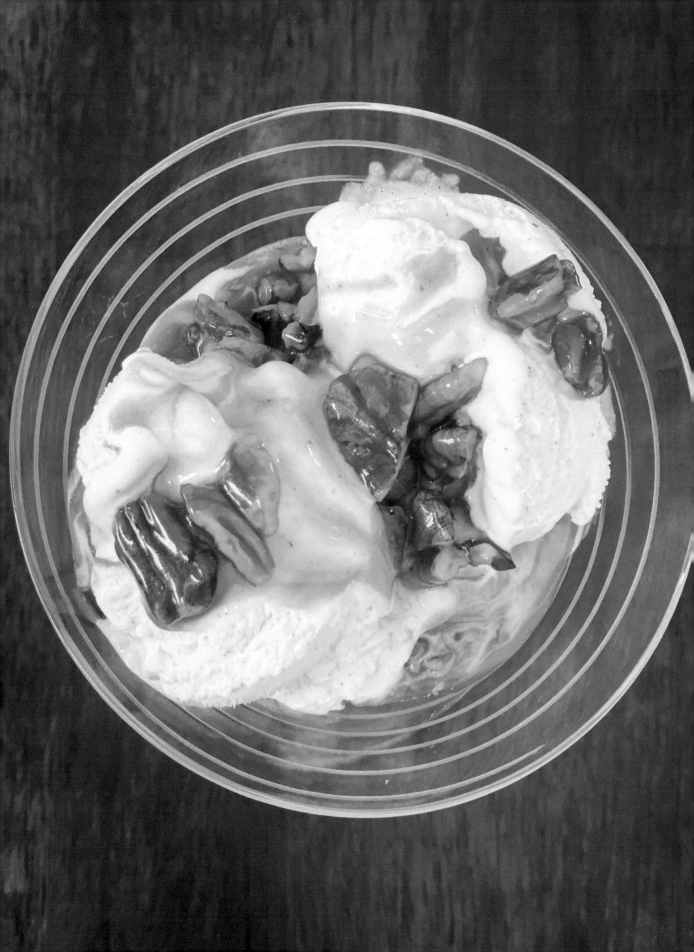

VANILLA BEAN ICE CREAM WITH BUTTERY BOURBON SAUCE

Ingredients

4 tablespoons butter

½ cup allulose

¼ cup powdered sweetener

2 cups heavy whipping cream

1 ½ teaspoons vanilla extract

3 vanilla beans, split and seeds scraped

2 eggs yolks, beaten

1 prepared batch of buttery bourbon sauce*

Directions

1. Heat a medium saucepan on medium heat.
2. Melt the butter with allulose and powdered sweetener. Stir in the heavy whipping cream, vanilla extract, and vanilla beans. Bring to a simmer.
3. In a separate bowl, add the 2 beaten egg yolks along with 2 tablespoons of the vanilla cream mixture and stir to temper.
4. Pour eggs into saucepan with cream mixture and whisk until combined.
5. Remove from heat, pour into a bowl, and refrigerate for 30 minutes.
6. Add chilled mixture to a 2-quart ice cream maker and churn according to your ice cream maker's instructions.
7. Scoop into a bowl and top with warm buttery bourbon sauce.

Pro Tip

Ice cream can be stored in the freezer for up to 2 weeks.

*Buttery bourbon sauce recipe on page 195.

WHIPPED & CREAMED

143

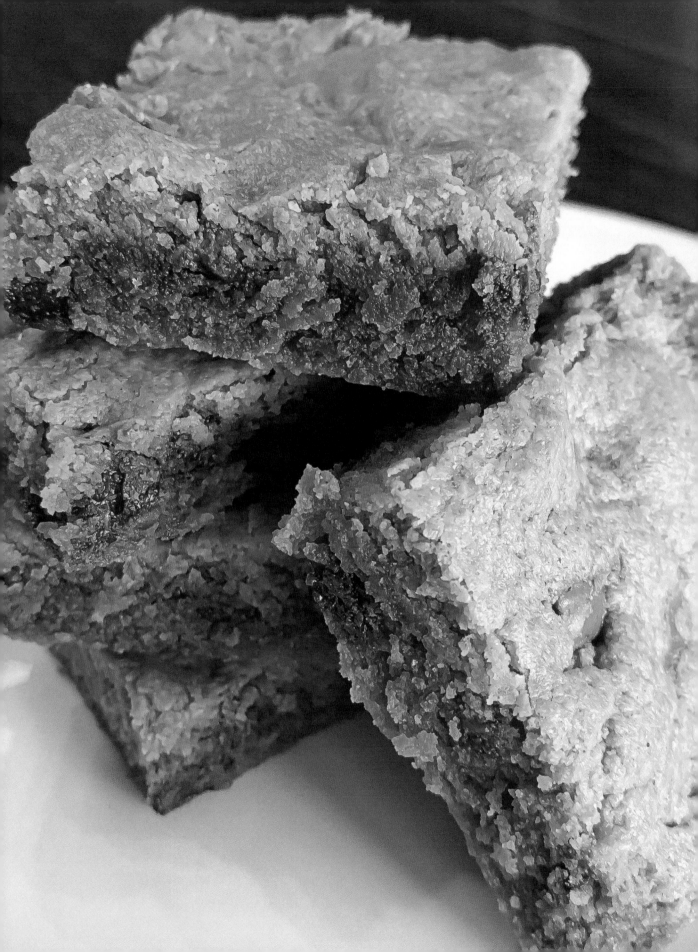

Prep Time: 15 minutes
Cook Time: 20 minutes
Yield: 9 servings

PEANUT BUTTER BLONDIES

Ingredients

1 cup almond flour
½ teaspoon baking soda
¼ teaspoon salt
½ cup creamy natural peanut butter
4 tablespoons butter, softened
½ cup powdered sweetener
2 eggs
1 teaspoon vanilla extract
½ cup no-sugar-added chocolate chips

Directions

1. Preheat oven to 325°F and grease an 8x8 baking dish.
2. In a medium mixing bowl, mix the almond flour, baking soda, and salt until combined.
3. In a separate bowl, use an electric hand mixer to beat together the peanut butter, butter, and powdered sweetener until smooth. Add in the eggs and vanilla and continue to beat.
4. Gradually mix in the almond flour. Once thoroughly combined, fold in the chocolate chips.
5. Pour mixture into the baking dish and bake for 16-20 minutes.
6. Remove from oven and allow to cool for 30 minutes before cutting.

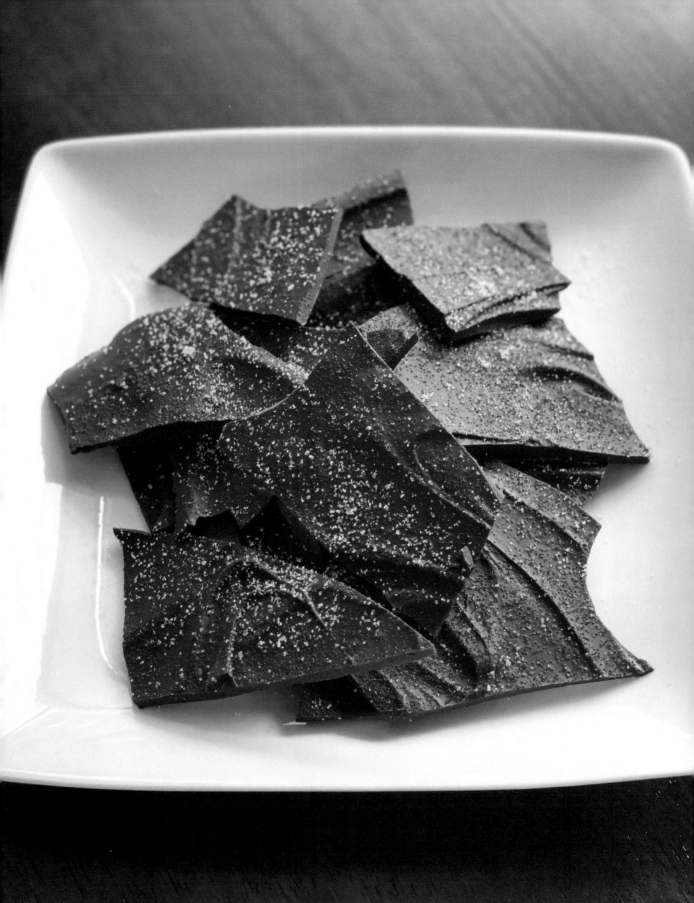

Prep Time: 10 minutes
Cook Time: 0 minutes
Yield: 8 servings

SWEET & SPICY MIDNIGHT BARK

Ingredients

1 8-ounce package of no-sugar-added dark chocolate chips (reserve 2 tablespoons for topping)

½ teaspoon cayenne pepper (more if you want it spicier)

2 tablespoons granular sweetener

2 tablespoons walnuts, chopped

Directions

1. In a microwave-safe bowl, melt chocolate chips in 30-second intervals, stirring in between. Stir in cayenne pepper.

2. Spread the chocolate mixture onto a baking sheet lined with parchment paper, careful not to spread too thin.

3. Add chopped walnuts, 2 tablespoons no-sugar-added chocolate chips, granular sweetener, and extra cayenne if desired.

4. Place the sheet in the freezer for 15-30 minutes.

5. Once the bark has hardened, break into pieces and enjoy.

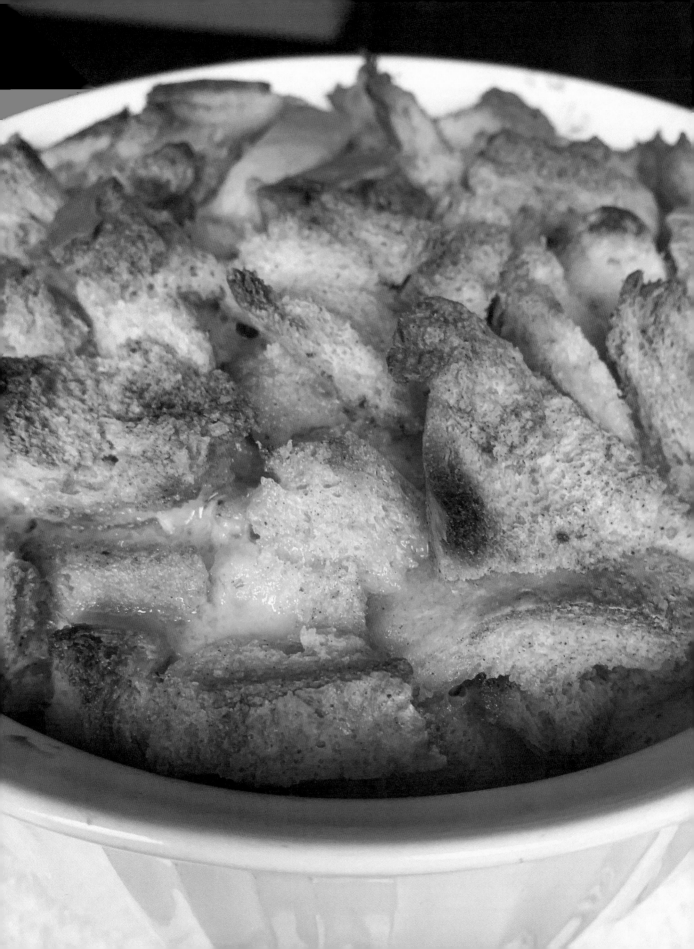

Prep Time: 15 minutes
Cook Time: 75 minutes
Yield: 12 servings

VANILLA RUM BREAD PUDDING

Ingredients

BREAD PUDDING

1 loaf low-carb bread*
1 ½ cups half & half
¾ cup granular sweetener
½ cup heavy whipping cream
4 eggs
¼ teaspoon salt
1 ½ teaspoons vanilla extract
1 ½ teaspoons ground cinnamon
butter for frying the bread

VANILLA RUM SAUCE

4 tablespoons butter
1 teaspoon vanilla extract
¼ cup powdered sweetener
½ cup heavy whipping cream
2 tablespoons dark rum

Directions

1. Preheat oven to 350°F and grease a 9x13 baking dish.
2. Cube the bread and place in a large frying pan on medium-high heat with 2 tablespoons melted butter. Fry the bread cubes until lightly golden with crisp edges. Remove from pan and place in the baking dish.
3. In a large mixing bowl, whisk together the half & half, granular sweetener, heavy whipping cream, eggs, salt, vanilla, and cinnamon. Pour over the top of the bread. Make sure to fill all the empty spaces.
4. Cover baking dish with plastic wrap and refrigerate for at least 4 hours. (Overnight is better)
5. Uncover and bake for 1 hour to 1 hour and 15 minutes until puffed and golden.
6. While baking, heat a small sauce pot on medium heat and whisk together all the ingredients for the vanilla rum sauce. Drizzle warm sauce over the bread pudding and serve.

*Find low-carb bread options on page xvi.

WHIPPED & CREAMED

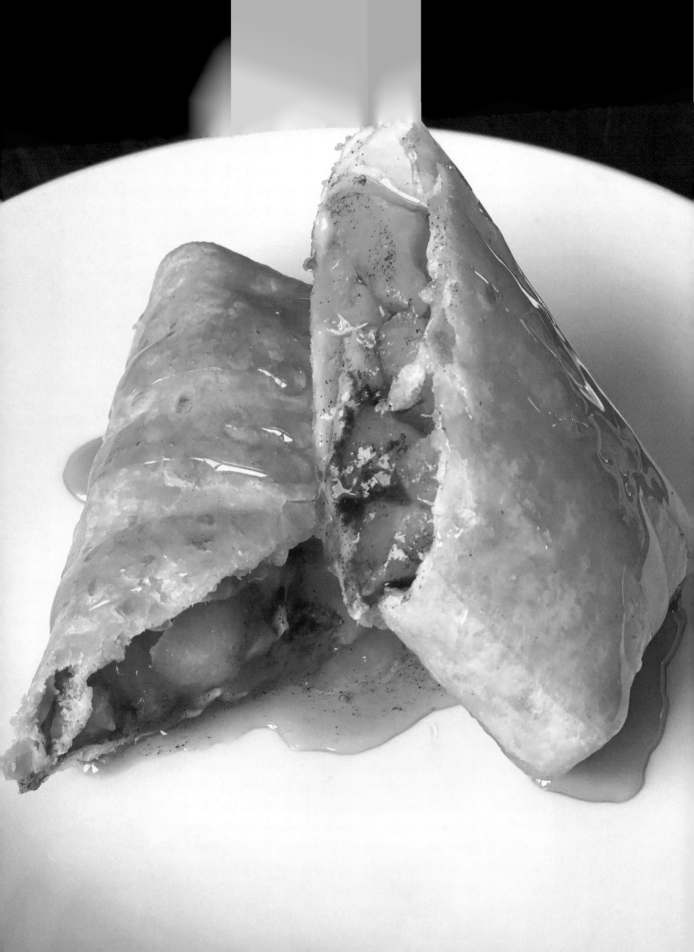

Prep Time: 40 minutes
Cook Time: 10 minutes
Yield: 6 servings

APPLE TURN-(ME)-OVER

Ingredients

4 chayotes
2 tablespoons butter
3 tablespoons Swerve brown sugar replacement
3 tablespoons sugar-free pancake syrup
1 teaspoon ground cinnamon
1 ½ teaspoons pumpkin pie spice
½ teaspoon xanthan gum
6 low-carb wraps*
Butter for frying

Directions

1. In a large pot of water, boil the chayotes whole with the skin on for 25-30 minutes, until fork tender. Allow to cool.
2. With a vegetable peeler, peel the skin. Slice length-wise and scoop out the seed with a spoon. Chop into small cubes and place in a bowl lined with paper towels to remove excess moisture. Set aside while you make the apple pie sauce.
3. Melt butter in a medium-sized pot. Add the brown sugar replacement and stir until dissolved. Add in the chayotes and mix to combine.
4. Stir in the rest of ingredients, except the xanthan gum, and simmer for 3 minutes while stirring.
5. At this time, add the xanthan gum if you feel you need to thicken the sauce more.
6. Remove from heat. Sauce will continue to thicken as it cools.
7. Taking a low-carb wrap, cut in half, length-wise, and fill each piece with cooled mixture. Fold to form a triangle.
8. In a large skillet, melt 2 tablespoons of butter. When hot, place the apple pies, seam side down, in the hot butter and cook until golden on both sides. Top with your favorite sugar-free caramel sauce, whipped cream, vanilla bean ice cream**, or sugar-free maple syrup.

Pro Tip

Use 10-15 drops of apple pie flavoring from One on One Flavors in the filling mixture.

*Find low-carb wrap options on page xvi.
**Vanilla bean ice cream recipe on page 143.

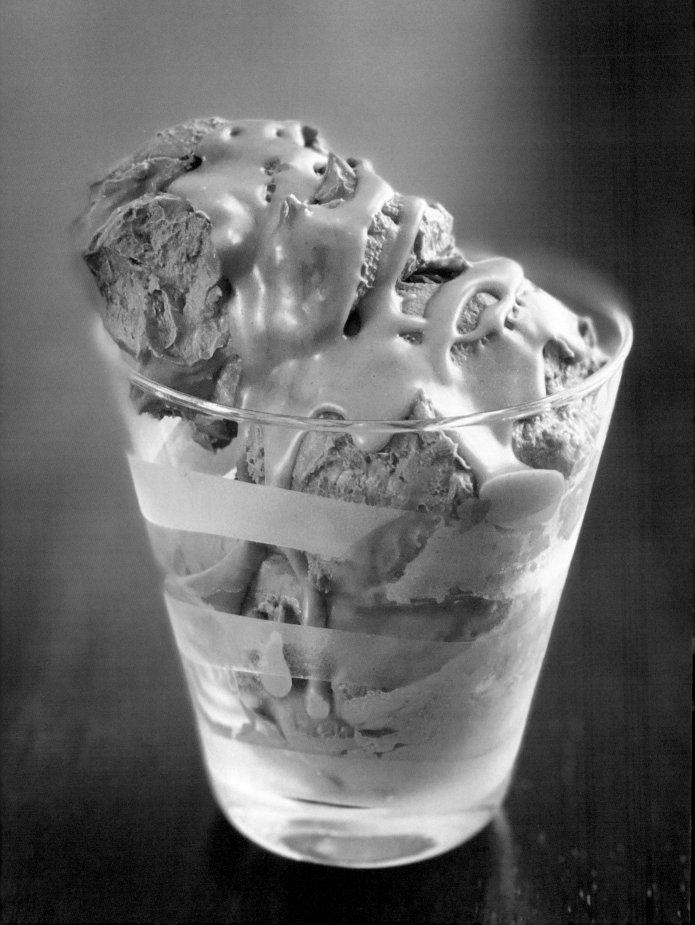

CHOCOLATE PEANUT BUTTER ICE CREAM

Ingredients

- 4 tablespoons butter
- ½ cup allulose
- ¼ cup powdered sweetener
- 2 cups heavy whipping cream
- 1 teaspoon vanilla extract
- 2 tablespoons sugar-free chocolate syrup
- 2 eggs yolks, beaten
- 3 heaping tablespoons unsweetened cocoa powder
- 3 tablespoons creamy natural peanut butter, melted

Directions

1. Heat a medium saucepan on medium heat.
2. Melt the butter with allulose and powdered sweetener. Stir in the heavy whipping cream, vanilla, and chocolate syrup until smooth. Bring to a simmer.
3. In a separate bowl, add the 2 beaten egg yolks along with 2 tablespoons of the chocolate mixture and stir to temper.
4. Pour eggs into saucepan with chocolate mixture and add cocoa powder. Whisk until combined.
5. Remove from heat, pour into a bowl, and refrigerate for 30 minutes.
6. Add cooled mixture to a 2-quart ice cream maker and churn according to your ice cream maker's instructions.
7. When done, keep churning while slowly pouring in the melted peanut butter.
8. Ice cream can be stored in the freezer for up to 2 weeks.

Pro Tip

Top with nuts and chopped sugar-free peanut butter cups.

WHIPPED & CREAMED

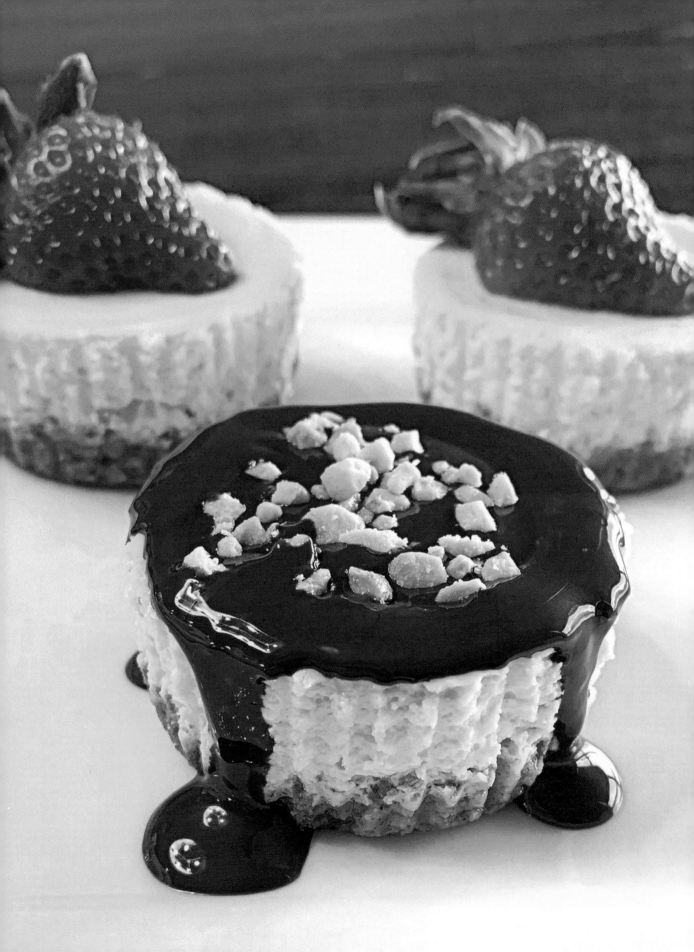

Prep Time: 10 minutes
Cook Time: 20 minutes
Yield: 12 servings

CHEESECAKE BITES

Ingredients

CRUST

¾ cup almond flour

⅓ cup walnuts

3 tablespoons butter, melted

¼ cup Swerve brown sugar replacement

¼ teaspoon salt

FILLING

1 8-ounce brick cream cheese, softened

⅓ cup powdered sweetener

¾ cup sour cream

½ teaspoon vanilla extract

¼ cup heavy whipping cream

Juice and zest of 1 lemon

1 egg plus 1 egg yolk, room temperature, slightly beaten

Directions

1. Preheat oven to 325°F and line cupcake pan with paper liners.
2. For the crust, pulse all ingredients in a food processor until combined and crumbly. Press mixture down into the bottoms on the cupcake cavities.
3. Bake mini crusts for 5 minutes and then set aside to work on the filling.
4. In a large mixing bowl, beat the softened cream cheese with an electric hand mixer until smooth and creamy. (Be careful not to over-beat and incorporate too much air.)
5. Add powdered sweetener and continue to mix.
6. Add in the sour cream, vanilla, heavy whipping cream, lemon juice, and lemon zest, beating until well-combined.
7. Turning the hand mixer on low speed, gradually add the slightly beaten eggs, mixing until just incorporated.
8. Evenly spoon the mixture into the cupcake cavities and bake for 20 minutes.
9. Remove from oven and allow to cool on the countertop for 1 hour. Store cheesecakes in the fridge.

Pro Tip

Top cheesecakes with fresh fruit or melted no-sugar-added chocolate chips.

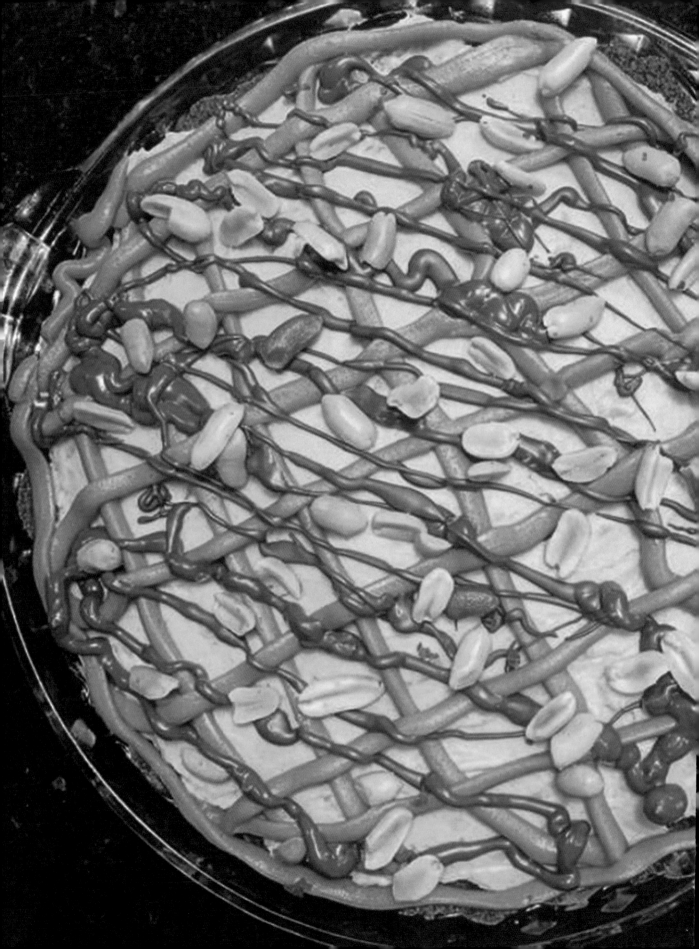

PEANUT BUTTER PIE

Ingredients

CRUST

6 tablespoons butter, melted

1 ¾ cups almond flour

⅓ cup granulated sweetener

3 tablespoons unsweetened cocoa powder

1 tablespoon instant espresso powder

FILLING

8 ounces mascarpone cheese, room temperature

⅔ cup creamy natural peanut butter

1 ¾ cup heavy whipping cream

½ teaspoon vanilla extract

¼ teaspoon xanthan gum

½ cup powdered sweetener

TOPPING

4 ounces no-sugar-added chocolate chips

3 tablespoons creamy natural peanut butter

1 tablespoon heavy whipping cream

1 tablespoon powdered sweetener

¼ cup salted peanuts, chopped

Directions

1. Preheat oven to 350°F and grease a 9-inch pie plate.
2. In a medium-sized mixing bowl, stir together melted butter, almond flour, granulated sweetener, cocoa powder, and espresso powder until thoroughly combined.
3. Press crust mixture into the bottom of the pie plate and up the sides. Bake for 10 minutes.
4. For the filling, stir together the mascarpone and peanut butter until creamy.
5. In a separate bowl, beat the heavy whipping cream, vanilla, xanthan gum, and powdered sweetener with an electric hand mixer until stiff peaks form.
6. Gently fold the peanut butter mixture into the whipped cream.
7. Spoon the filling into the pie crust and smooth the top.
8. Chill in the freezer for 25 minutes.
9. To prepare the topping, stir together the peanut butter, heavy whipping cream, and powdered sweetener. Spoon mixture into a piping bag and pipe the peanut butter over the top of the pie.
10. In a microwave-safe bowl, heat the chocolate in 30-second intervals, stirring in between, until melted. Drizzle the chocolate over the pie and then sprinkle with chopped peanuts.
11. Store in fridge for a creamier pie or the freezer for a firmer pie.

WHIPPED & CREAMED

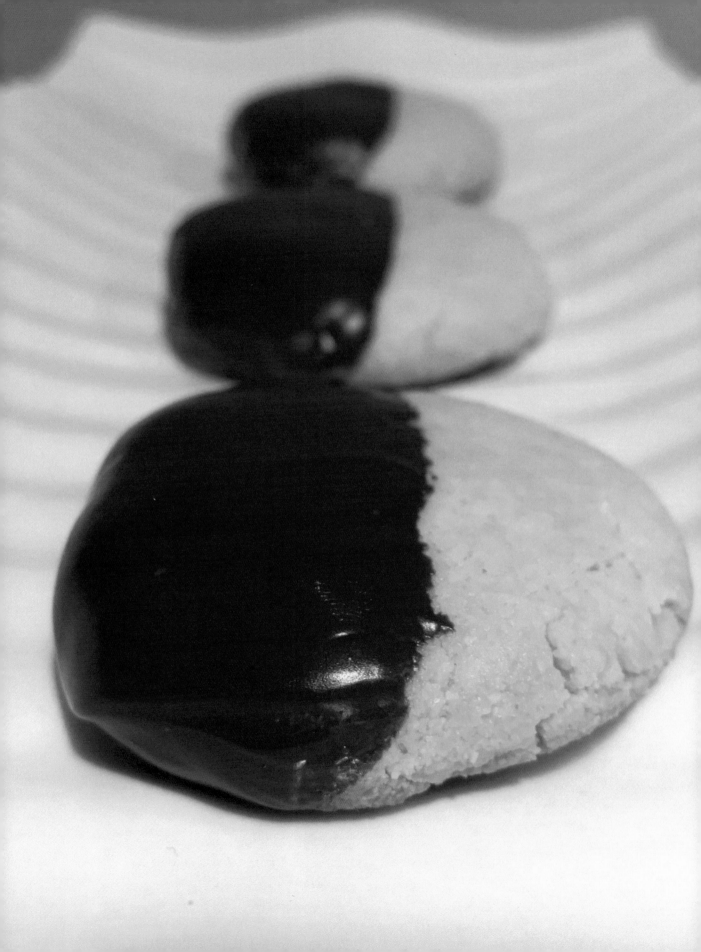

Prep Time: 10 minutes
Cook Time: 12 minutes
Yield: 12 servings

TUXEDO SHORTBREAD COOKIES

 Ingredients

 Directions

SHORTBREAD

2 ½ cups almond flour
¼ cup granular sweetener
Pinch of salt
6 tablespoons butter, room temperature
1 teaspoon vanilla extract

CHOCOLATE DIP

½ cup no-sugar-added chocolate chips
1 teaspoon coconut oil

1. Preheat oven to 350°F and line a cookie sheet with parchment paper.
2. Cream the butter and granular sweetener with an electric hand mixer until fluffy. Mix in the vanilla extract.
3. While beating, slowly add the almond flour a ½ cup at a time. Dough will be slightly crumbly.
4. Roll dough into balls, place on the cookie sheet, and then flatten the dough slightly.
5. Bake for 11-13 minutes until the edges start to golden. Remove from oven and allow to fully cool before handling.
6. For the chocolate dip, melt chocolate and coconut oil in a small microwave-safe bowl in 30-second intervals, stirring in between.
7. Once cookies have completely cools, dip ½ of the cookie into the chocolate and return to the parchment paper. Chill cookies in the refrigerator for 10-15 to allow the chocolate to set.

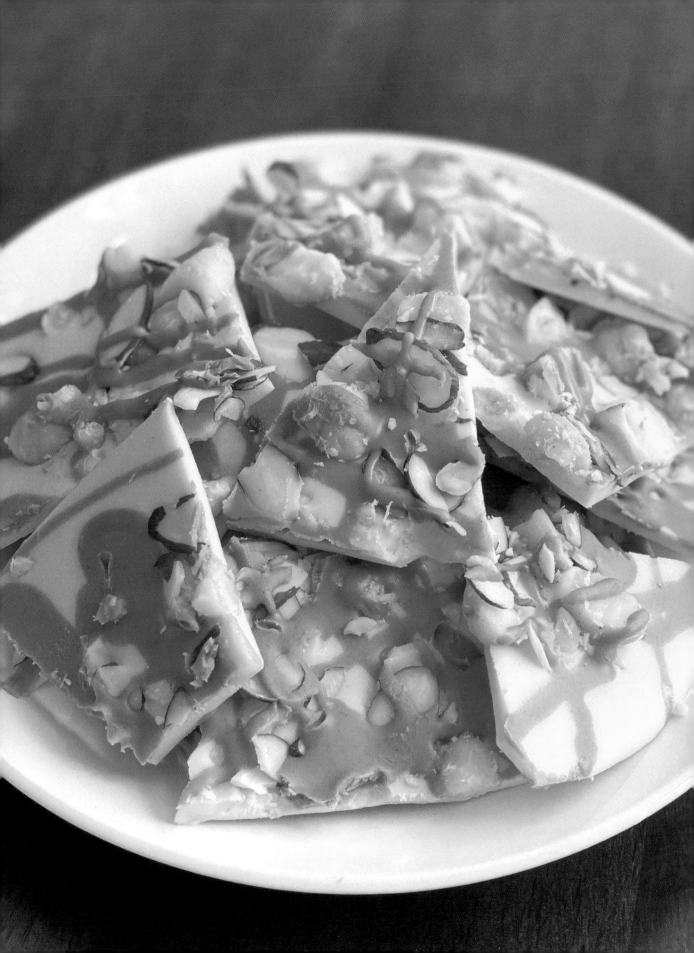

Prep Time: 10 minutes
Cook Time: 0 minutes
Yield: 8 servings

WHITE CHOCOLATE PEANUT BUTTER BARK

Ingredients

1 bag no-sugar-added white chocolate chips
2 tablespoons creamy natural peanut butter
¼ cup almonds, chopped
¼ cup macadamia nuts, chopped

Directions

1. In a microwave-safe bowl, heat the white chocolate chips in 30 second intervals, stirring in between, until completely melted.
2. Pour white chocolate onto a baking sheet lined with parchment paper and spread into an even layer.
3. Melt peanut butter in the microwave for 20 seconds and immediately pour over the white chocolate.
4. Swirl the peanut butter throughout the white chocolate using a toothpick.
5. Before the white chocolate and peanut butter cools completely, sprinkle the chopped nuts over the top and gently press into the chocolate so they stick.
6. Place baking sheet into the freezer 20 minutes or until bark has fully harden.
7. Break bark into pieces and enjoy.

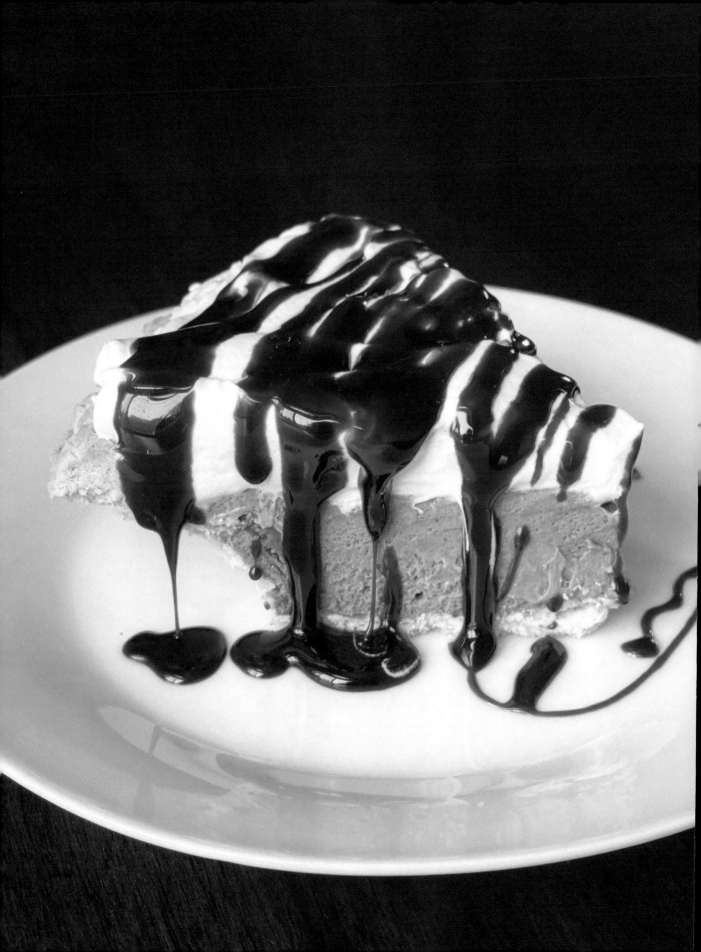

Prep Time: 15 minutes
Cook Time: 23 minutes
Yield: 8 servings

FRENCH SILK PIE

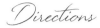

Ingredients

CRUST

1 ½ cups almond flour

4 tablespoons butter

½ teaspoon salt

1 ounce cream cheese

1 teaspoon apple cider vinegar

1 egg

FILLING

16 ounces cream cheese, room temperature

4 tablespoons sour cream

4 tablespoons butter

1 tablespoon vanilla extract

½ cup powdered sweetener

½ cup cocoa powder

WHIPPED TOPPING

1 cup whipping cream

2 teaspoons powdered sweetener

1 teaspoon vanilla extract

Directions

1. Preheat oven to 350°F and grease a 9-inch pie plate.
2. In a food processor, blend almond flour, butter, salt, and cream cheese until coarse and crumbly. Add in apple cider vinegar and egg and mix again until fully incorporated.
3. Roll dough into a ball, cover in plastic wrap, and chill for 2 hours in the refrigerator.
4. Press the dough into the bottom of the pie plate and up the sides before piercing with a fork. Dough will be sticky.
5. Bake crust for 15 minutes. Remove from oven, loosely cover the edges with foil, and continue to bake for an additional 7-10 minutes until golden.
6. For the filling, use an electric hand mixer and beat together the cream cheese, sour cream, butter, vanilla extract, powdered sweetener, and cocoa powder in a medium bowl until fluffy.
7. In a separate bowl, pour in the heavy whipped cream and beat with electric hand mixer until soft peaks form. Add in the powdered sweetener and vanilla and continue to beat until stiff peaks form.
8. With a rubber spatula, gently fold in the whipped cream, 1 cup at a time, into the chocolate cream mixture, careful not to break down the fluffiness of the whipped cream.
9. Spoon the filling into the completely cooled pie crust and smooth out the top. Cover and refrigerate for 2 hours before serving.

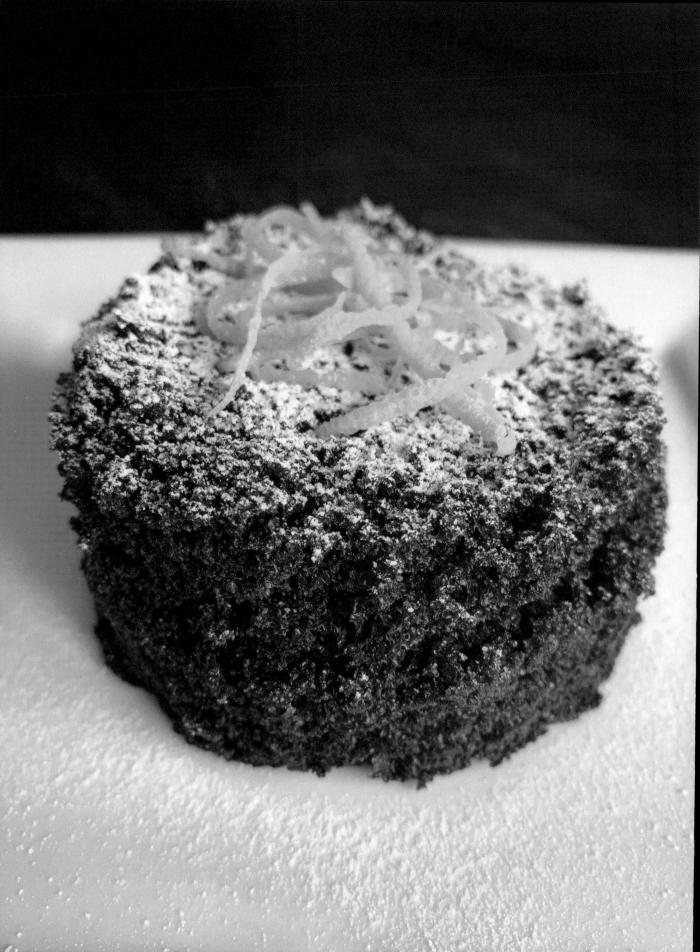

Prep Time: 3 minutes
Cook Time: 90 seconds
Yield: 1 serving

CHOCOLATE ORANGE MUG CAKE

Ingredients

- 1 tablespoon butter
- 3 tablespoons almond flour
- ½ teaspoon baking powder
- 1 tablespoon unsweetened cocoa powder
- ½ teaspoon orange extract or 1 teaspoon fresh orange zest
- 2 tablespoons granular sweetener
- 1 egg

Directions

1. In a large mug or ramekin, melt butter in the microwave.
2. Add in the remaining ingredients and stir with a fork until fully combined.
3. Microwave for 90 seconds until set and fluffy.

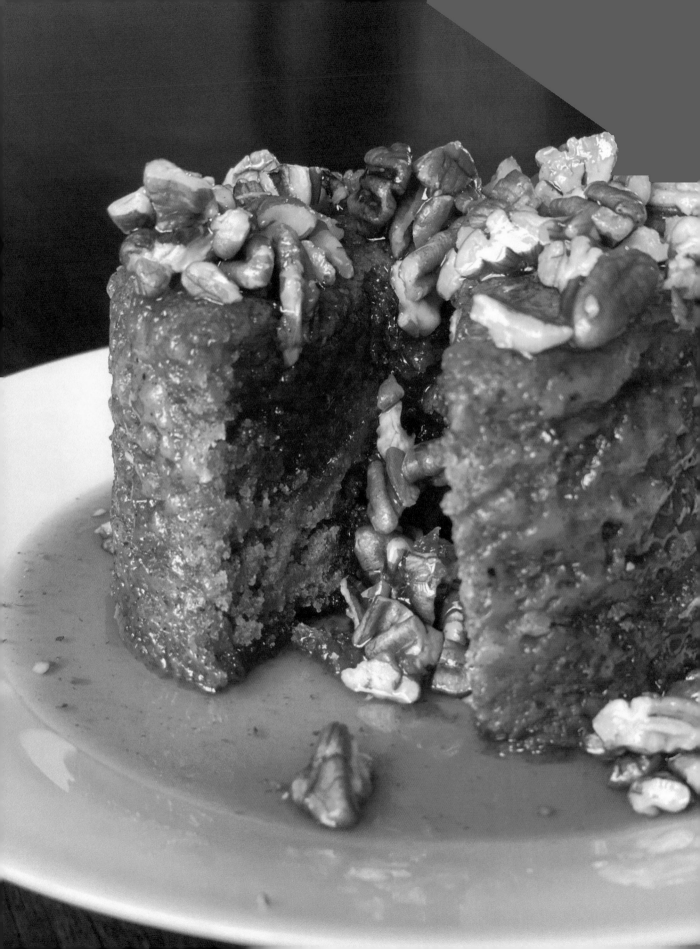

Prep Time: 5 minutes
Cook Time: 90 seconds
Yield: 1 serving

MAPLE PECAN SPICE MUG CAKE

Ingredients

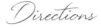

Directions

1 tablespoon butter

3 tablespoons almond flour

1 tablespoon granulated sweetener

¼ teaspoon cinnamon

⅛ teaspoon pumpkin pie seasoning

¼ teaspoon molasses

⅛ teaspoon vanilla extract

1 egg

MAPLE PECAN TOPPING

1 tablespoon butter

2 tablespoons powdered sweetener

2 teaspoons sugar-free pancake syrup

1 tablespoon pecans, chopped

⅛ teaspoon maple extract (optional)

1. In a large mug or ramekin, melt butter in the microwave.
2. Add in the remaining ingredients and stir with a fork until fully combined.
3. Microwave for 90 seconds until set and fluffy.
4. For the topping, melt butter in a small, microwave-safe bowl. Stir in powdered sweetener, pancake syrup, and maple extract (optional) with a fork until smooth.
5. Mix in pecans and microwave for an additional 20 seconds. Pour over warm cake and enjoy.

WHIPPED & CREAMED

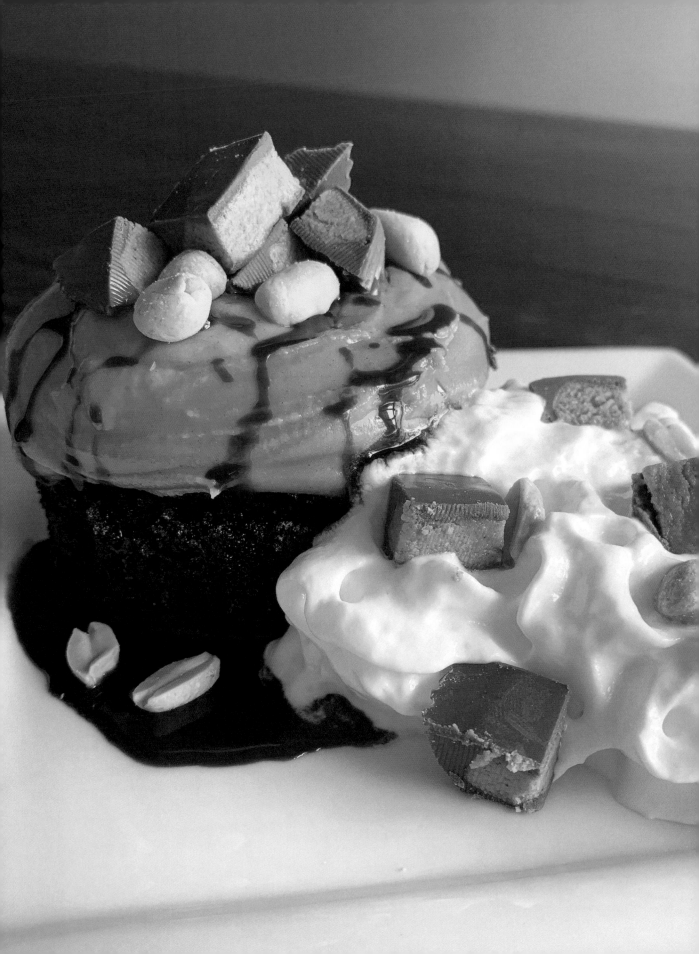

Prep Time: 3 minutes
Cook Time: 90 seconds
Yield: 1 serving

CHOCOLATE PEANUT BUTTER MUG CAKE

Ingredients

1 tablespoon butter
1 tablespoon creamy natural peanut butter
3 tablespoons almond flour
½ teaspoon baking powder
1 tablespoon unsweetened cocoa powder
2 tablespoons granular sweetener
1 egg
Pinch of salt

Directions

1. In a large mug or ramekin, melt butter and peanut butter in the microwave.
2. Add in the remaining ingredients and stir with a fork until fully combined.
3. Microwave for 90 seconds until set and fluffy.

Pro Tip

Melt extra peanut butter to drizzle over the top, add chopped sugar-free peanut butter cups, or top with whipped cream.

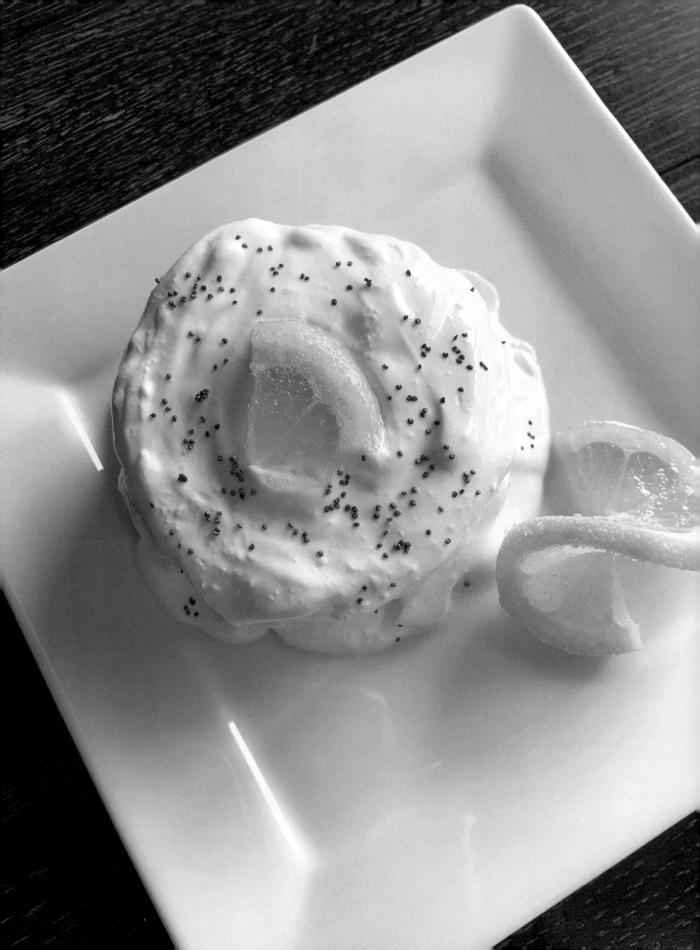

LEMON POPPY SEED MUG CAKE

Ingredients

2 tablespoons butter

3 tablespoons almond flour

1 tablespoon coconut flour

1 ½ tablespoons granular sweetener

¼ teaspoon baking powder

¼ teaspoon poppy seeds

1 teaspoon lemon zest

1 teaspoon lemon juice

1 tablespoon heavy whipping cream

⅛ teaspoon almond extract

1 egg

GLAZE

2 tablespoons powdered sweetener

1 teaspoon lemon juice

1 teaspoon heavy whipping cream

Directions

1. In a large mug or ramekin, melt butter in the microwave.

2. Using a fork, stir in the heavy whipping cream, lemon juice, almond extract, and egg until combined. Add in almond flour, coconut flour, granular sweetener, baking powder, poppy seeds, and lemon zest and mix together.

3. Microwave for 2 minutes, until set and fluffy.

4. For the glaze, whisk together all the ingredients and drizzle over the warm cake.

WHIPPED & CREAMED

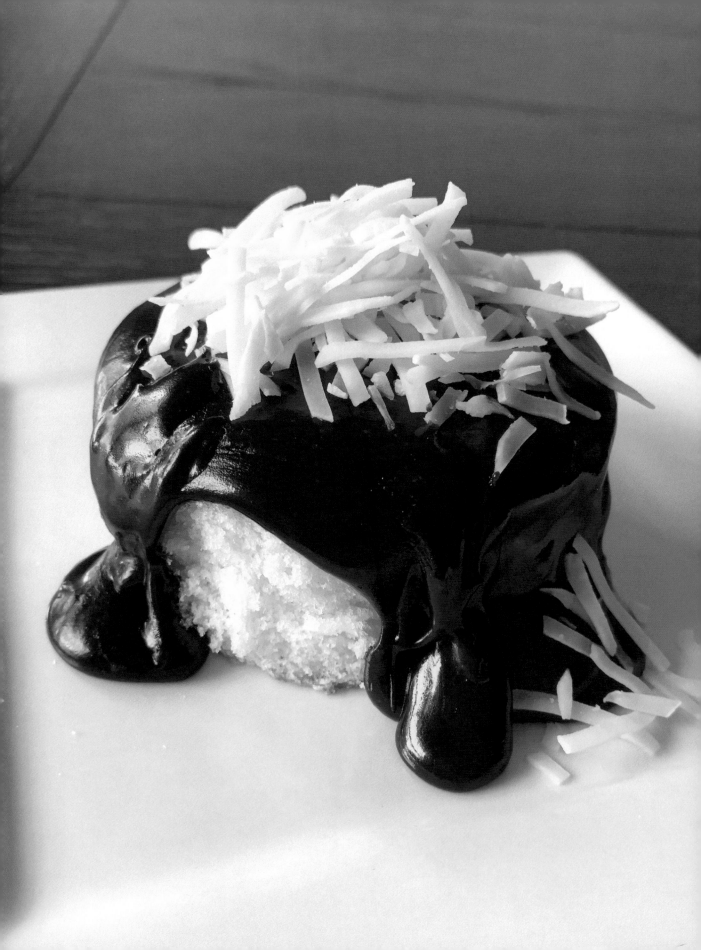

COCOA BUNNY MUG CAKE

Ingredients

1 tablespoon butter
2 tablespoons coconut flour
¼ teaspoon baking powder
1 tablespoon granular sweetener
2 tablespoons half & half
⅛ teaspoon almond extract
½ tablespoon unsweetened shredded coconut
1 tablespoon no-sugar-added chocolate chips

Directions

1. In a large mug or ramekin, melt butter in the microwave.
11. Add in the remaining ingredients and stir with a fork until fully combined.
12. Microwave for 90 seconds until set and fluffy.

Pro Tip

Melt 2 tablespoons of no-sugar-added chocolate chips with 1 teaspoon coconut oil in the microwave and drizzle over the warm cake with a light sprinkling of unsweetened shredded coconut.

WHIPPED & CREAMED

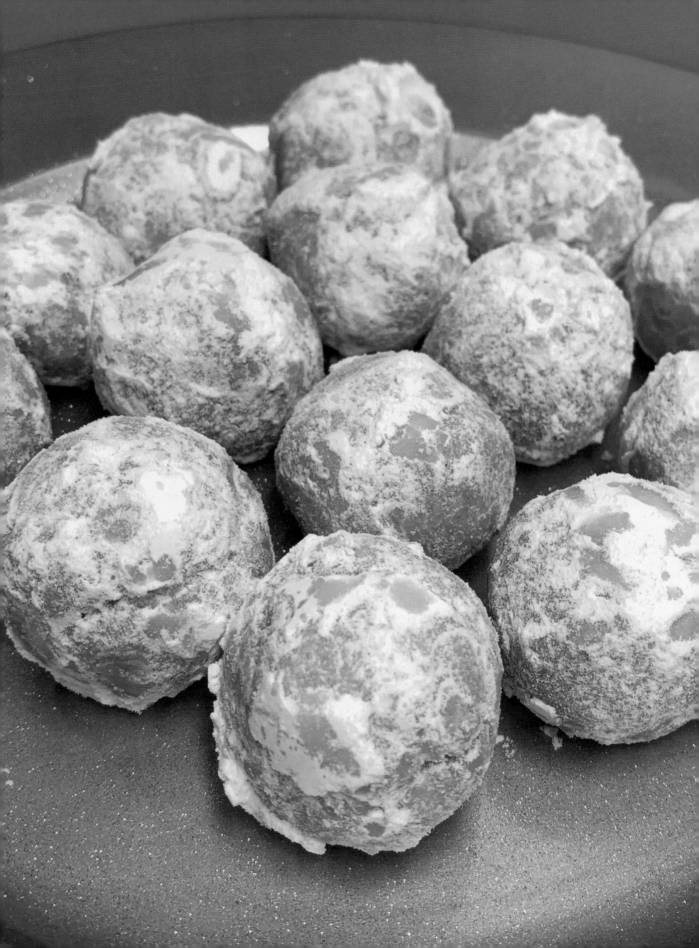

Prep Time: 15 minutes
Cook Time: 18 minutes
Yield: 12 servings

RUSSIAN TEA CAKES

Ingredients

1 cup walnuts

1 ½ cups almond flour

8 tablespoons cold butter, cubed

1 teaspoon vanilla

½ cup powdered sweetener + ¼ cup for cookie
   topping

1 egg

Pinch of salt

Directions

1. Preheat oven to 350°F and line baking sheet with parchment paper.
2. Using a large food processor, pulse walnuts a few times to chop.
3. Add remaining ingredients and continue to pulse until the dough forms.
4. Roll dough into 18-20 balls and place on baking sheet and chill in the freezer for 25 minutes.
5. Bake for 15-18 minutes until lightly golden.
6. Allow to cool for 5 minutes and then gently roll the warm cookies in the remaining ¼ cup of powdered sugar. Warm cookies will be very delicate, so handle with care. Let the cookies fully cool for 30 minutes so they can properly set before eating.

Pro Tip

Try adding ½ teaspoon of lemon extract or 1 teaspoon of fresh lemon juice for a little zing!

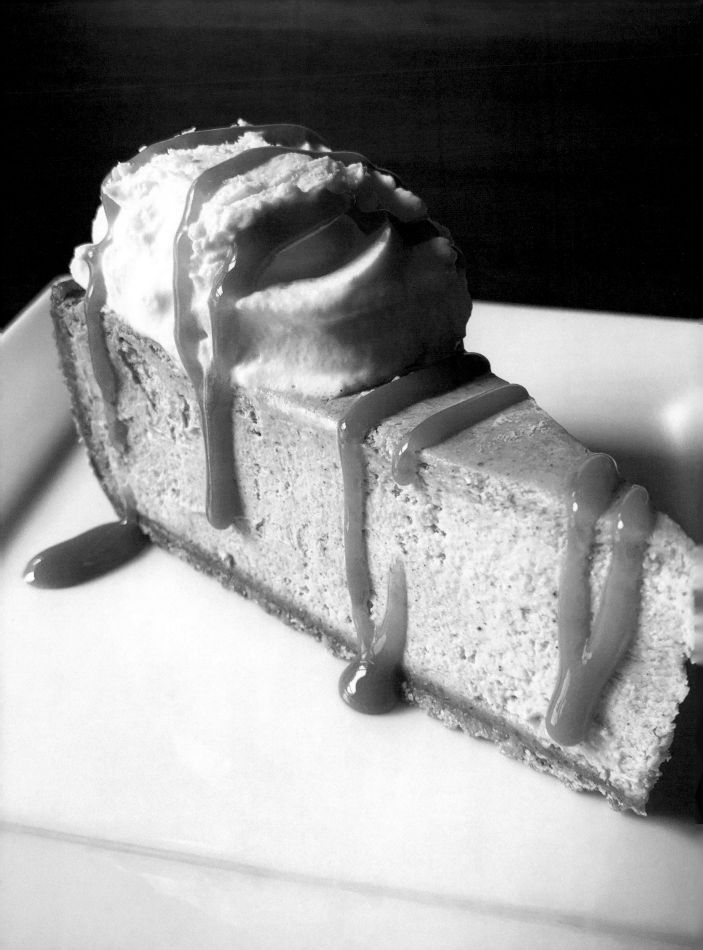

Prep Time: 20 minutes
Cook Time: 60 minutes
Yield: 10 servings

DRUNKEN PUMPKIN CHEESECAKE

Ingredients

CRUST

6 tablespoons butter, melted

2 cups almond flour

¼ cup walnuts

⅓ cup granular sweetener

Pinch of salt

FILLING

32 ounces brick cream cheese, softened (4 bricks)

1 ⅓ cups powdered sweetener

1cup sour cream

1 tablespoon pumpkin pie spice

1 ⅓ cups pure pumpkin puree

2 teaspoons vanilla extract

2 tablespoons + 2 teaspoons brandy liquor

2 eggs

Pro Tip

Top with whipped cream or drizzle salted caramel sauce* over the top.

*Salted caramel sauce recipe on page 193.

Directions

1. Preheat oven to 350°F and start a large pot of boiling water for the water bath.
2. For the crust, pulse all ingredients in a food processor until combined and crumbly. Press mixture down into the bottom of a 10-inch spring form pan and about halfway up the sides.
3. Bake for 5 minutes and then set aside.
4. For the filling, use a large mixing bowl and beat the softened cream cheese with an electric hand mixer until smooth and creamy. (Be careful not to over-beat and incorporate too much air.)
5. Add powdered sweetener and continue to mix.
6. Add in the sour cream, pumpkin pie spice, pumpkin puree, vanilla, and brandy, beating until well-combined.
7. Turning the hand mixer on low speed, add the egg, mixing until just incorporated.
8. Pour filling over the crust. Place the spring form pan down into a larger pan and place in the oven on the middle rack.
9. Fill the larger pan with boiling water until it's halfway up the sides of the spring form pan.
10. Bake for 1 hour. After an hour, turn the oven off and leave it in for another hour. Do not open the oven door during this process.
11. Remove from oven and allow to cool on the countertop for 30 minutes before storing in the fridge.

LET'S GE

Taco Seasoning

Basil, Parmesan, Parsley
Butter

Country Gravy

Beer Cheese

Sriracha Sauce

T SAUCY

Bang Bang Sauce

Shishido Pepper Sauce

Everyday Ranch

Salted Caramel Sauce

Buttery Bourbon Sauce

Sweetened Condensed Milk

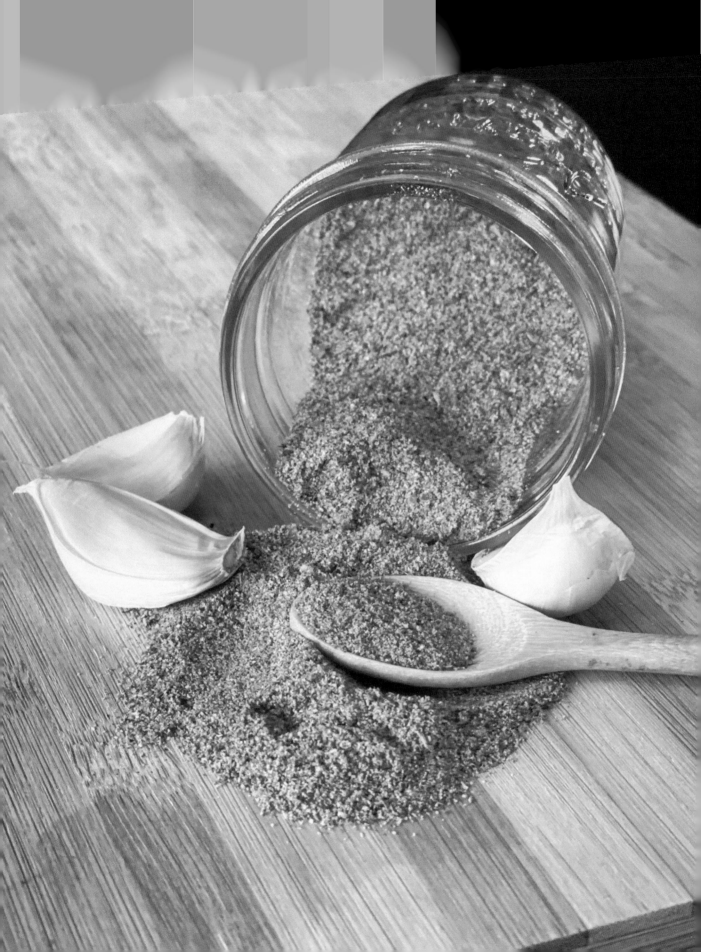

Prep Time: 5 minutes
Cook Time: 0 minutes
Yield: 1 serving

TACO SEASONING

Ingredients

½ teaspoon onion powder.
½ teaspoon garlic powder
1 tablespoon chili powder
1 teaspoon black pepper
1 tablespoon salt
1 ½ teaspoons ground cumin
½ teaspoon smoked paprika
½ teaspoon dried oregano

Directions

1. In a small bowl, stir together all the ingredients
2. Store in an airtight container.

Pro Tip

Triple the recipe to keep on-hand for when you make tacos or fajitas.

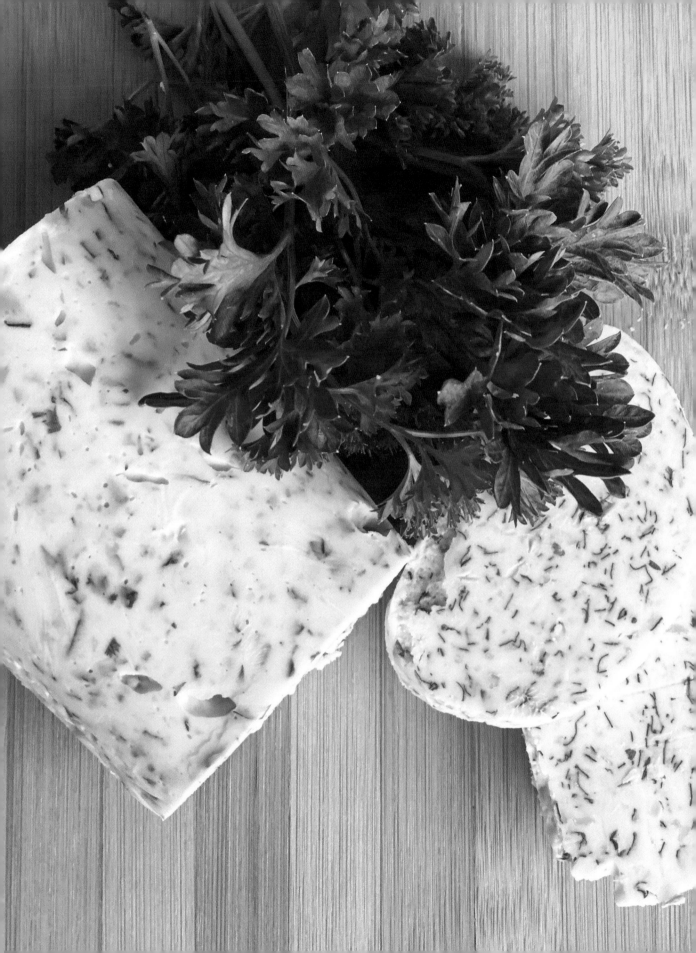

BASIL, PARMESAN, AND PARSLEY BUTTER

Ingredients

8 tablespoons butter, room temperature
¼ cup grated parmesan cheese
1 teaspoon dried basil
1 teaspoon dried parsley

Directions

1. In a small mixing bowl, add all the ingredients and use the back of a fork to smash all the ingredients together.
2. Once all the ingredients are thoroughly combined, wrap butter in plastic wrap and form into a log, securing the ends by twisting.
3. Chill the butter in the refrigerator for 1-4 hours.

Pro Tip

Serve on top of steak or use to cook veggies in.

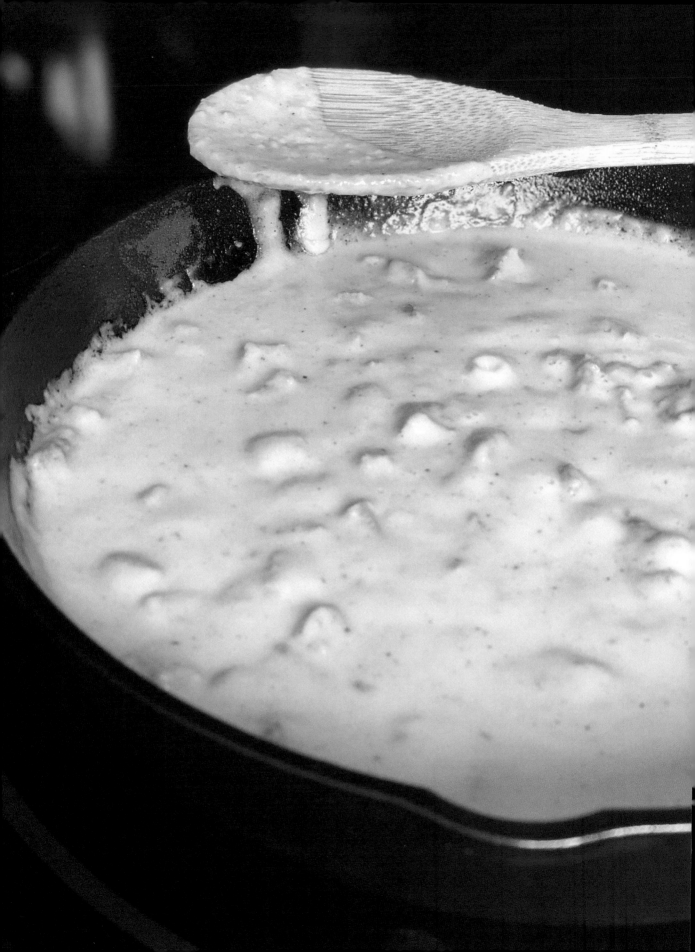

Prep Time: 5 minutes
Cook Time: 20 minutes
Yield: 6 servings

COUNTRY GRAVY

Ingredients

1 pound ground sausage
2 ounces cream cheese
½ cup heavy cream
1 teaspoon salt
½ teaspoon pepper
1 teaspoon onion powder
1 teaspoon garlic powder
Parsley for garnish

Directions

1. In a large skillet, brown the sausage meat and drain excess grease.
2. Add the cream cheese and melt before whisking in the heavy whipping cream, salt, pepper, onion powder, and garlic powder.
3. Allow to simmer for 5 minutes to marry the flavors.

Pro Tip

Serve on top of warm biscuits or fried chicken*.

*Fried chicken recipe on page 105.

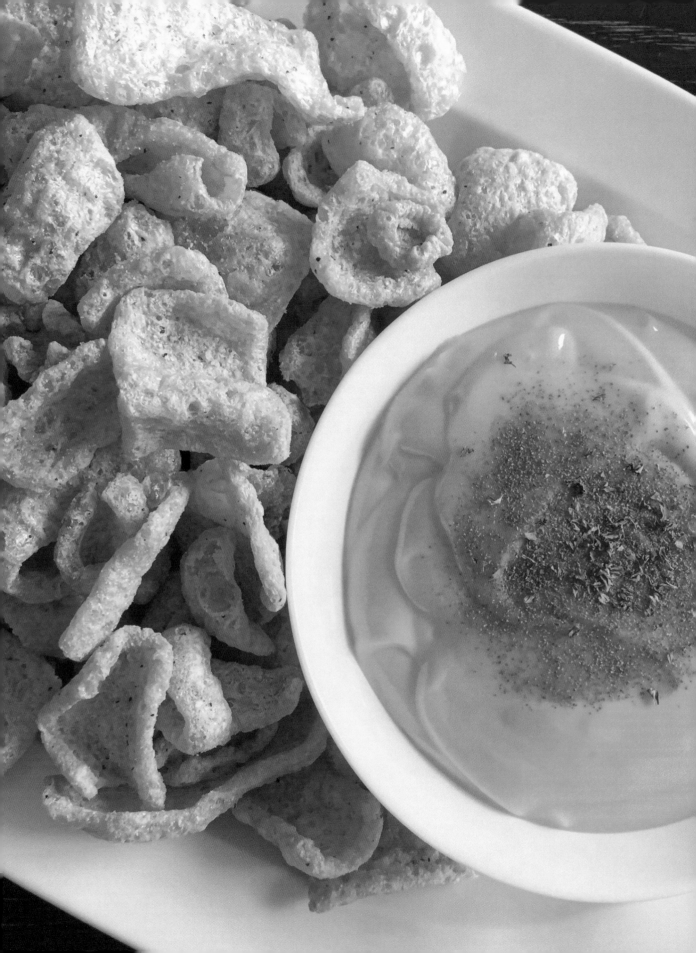

Prep Time: 3 minutes
Cook Time: 15 minutes
Yield: 16 servings
(2 tablespoons each)

BEER CHEESE

Ingredients

2 tablespoons butter

1 cup low-carb beer

1 teaspoon mustard

½ teaspoon paprika

Ground cayenne pepper to taste

¼ cup heavy whipping cream

2 ounces cream cheese

2 cups shredded cheddar cheese

Directions

1. In a medium saucepan, whisk together the butter, low-carb beer, mustard, paprika, and cayenne pepper. Bring to a boil.
2. Turn down the heat and simmer for 10 minutes while occasionally stirring.
3. Add in the cream cheese, heavy whipping cream, and cheddar cheese, stirring until combined and melted. Continue to cook for an additional 5 minutes while stirring.
4. Remove from heat and enjoy!

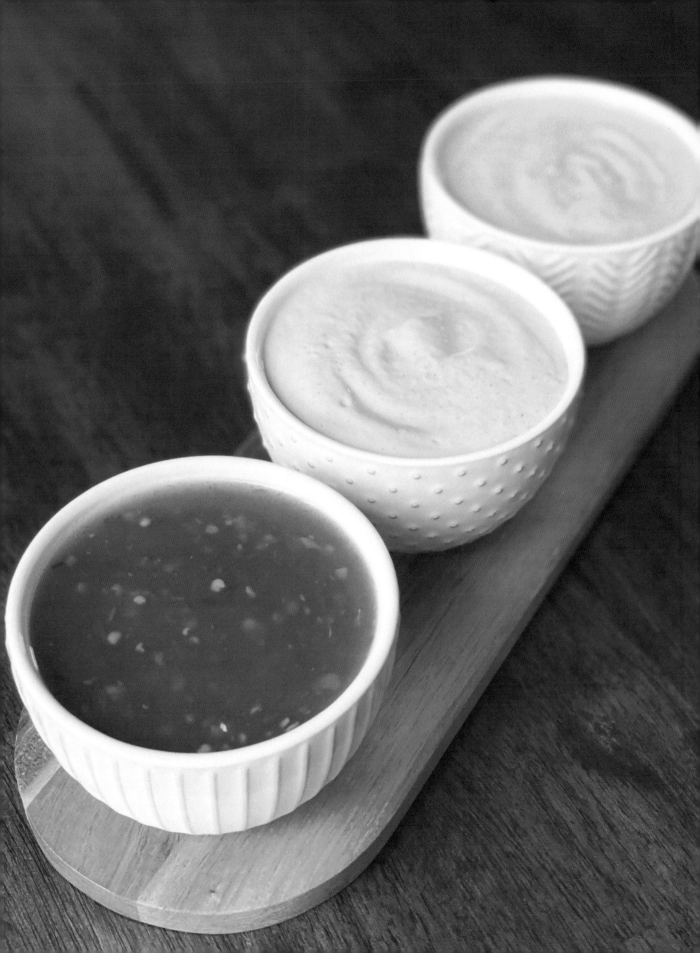

Prep Time: 3-6 minutes
Cook Time: 0-8 minutes
Yield: 4-8 servings

SAUCY THREESOME

SRIRACHA SAUCE

Ingredients

¼ cup sriracha chili sauce
¼ cup mayo
¼ cup sour cream
1 tablespoon powdered sweetener

Directions

1. Add all the ingredients to a mixing bowl and whisk to combine.

BANG BANG SAUCE

Ingredients

½ cup rice wine vinegar
½ cup water
½ cup granular sweetener
3 teaspoons red pepper flakes
1 teaspoon garlic powder
½ teaspoon salt
½ teaspoon xanthan gum

Directions

1. In a medium saucepan, add all ingredients, except xanthan gum, and bring to a boil.
2. Boil for 5 minutes while stirring to reduce mixture.
3. Remove from heat and stir in xanthan gum.
4. Allow mixture to thicken as it cools.

SHISHIDO PEPPER SAUCE

Ingredients

10 shishido peppers
½ cup sour cream
½ cup mayo
1 teaspoon minced garlic
2 jalapeños
1 teaspoon onion powder
1 teaspoon chili powder
½ teaspoon salt
1 teaspoon apple cider vinegar

Directions

1. Blister the peppers by placing them, whole, in a dry pan on medium-high heat until charred.
2. Remove from heat and allow to cool while you deseed the jalapeños.
3. When the shishido peppers have cooled cut the stems and discard.
4. In a food processor, add all the ingredients and blend until smooth.
5. You can enjoy right away or allow flavors to develop in the refrigerator for 1-2 hours. Store in an airtight container for up to a week.

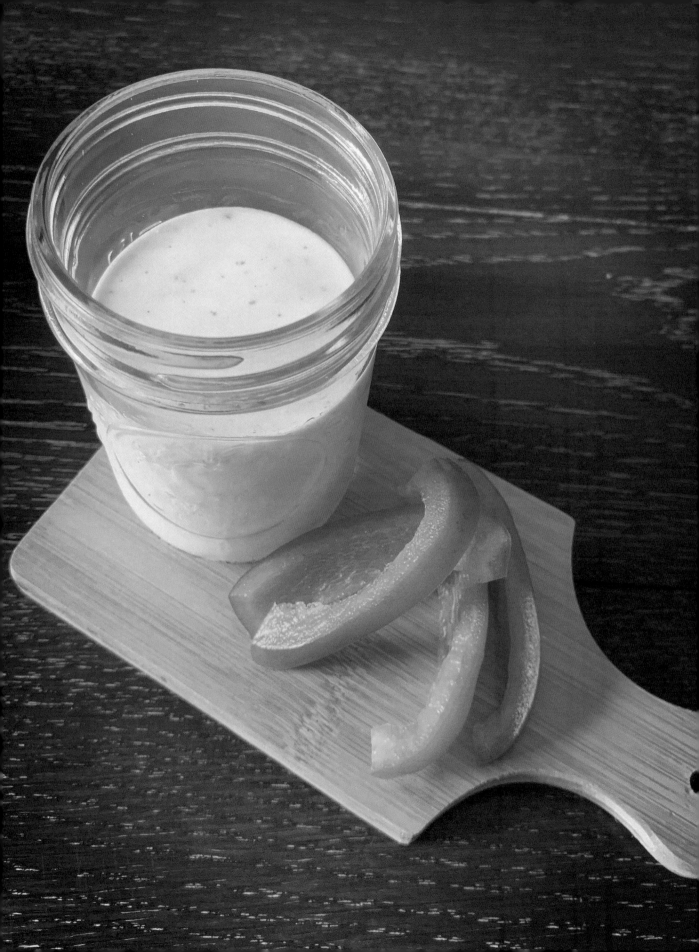

Prep Time: 5 minutes
Cook Time: 0 minutes
Yield: 10 servings

EVERYDAY RANCH

Ingredients

½ cup half & half
½ cup mayo
1 cup sour cream
2 tablespoons lemon juice (fresh if possible)
1 teaspoon dried dill
1 teaspoon dried chives
2 tablespoons dried parsley
1 teaspoon garlic powder
1 teaspoon onion powder
½ teaspoon salt
¼ teaspoon pepper

Directions

1. Add all the ingredients, except the half & half, to a medium-sized mixing bowl and stir.
2. Slowly add the half & half until you reach your desired consistency.
3. Chill in the refrigerator for 1 hour.

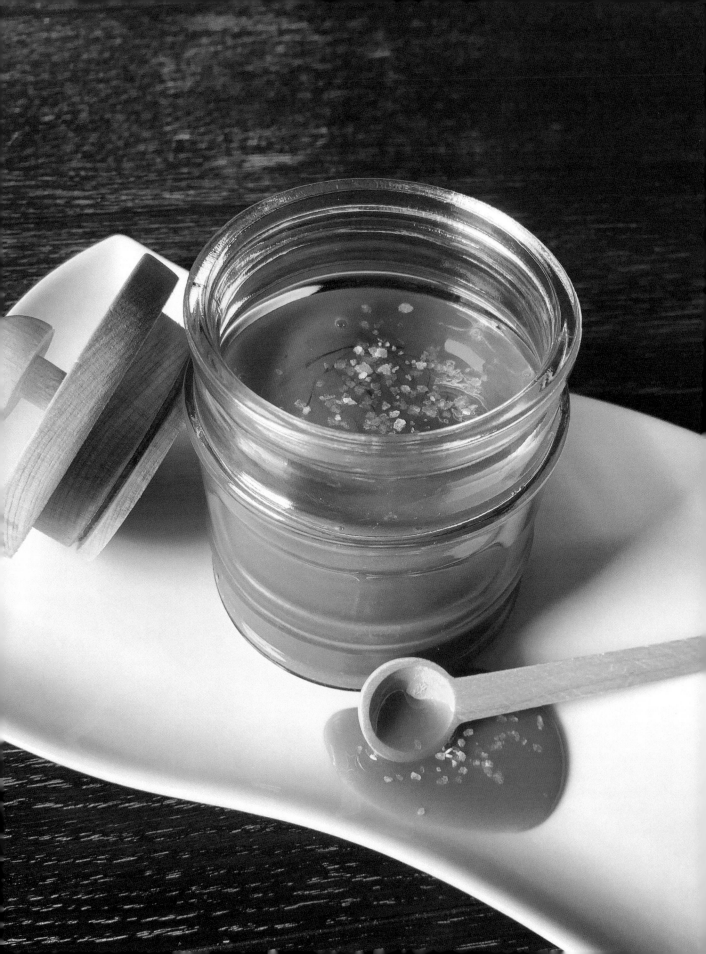

SALTED CARAMEL SAUCE

Ingredients

5 tablespoons butter
¼ cup Swerve brown sugar replacement
⅔ cup heavy whipping cream
1 teaspoon vanilla extract
½ teaspoon salt

Directions

1. In a small saucepan on medium-low heat, add the butter and brown it. This will take roughly 7-10 minutes for it to reach a deep golden color.
2. Whisk in the remaining ingredients, and continue to cook for an additional 7-10 minutes, stirring occasionally, until the sauce thickens.
3. Once cooled, store in a glass container in the refrigerator.

Pro Tip

Caramel might solidify in the fridge. If this happens, microwave for 20 seconds and stir.

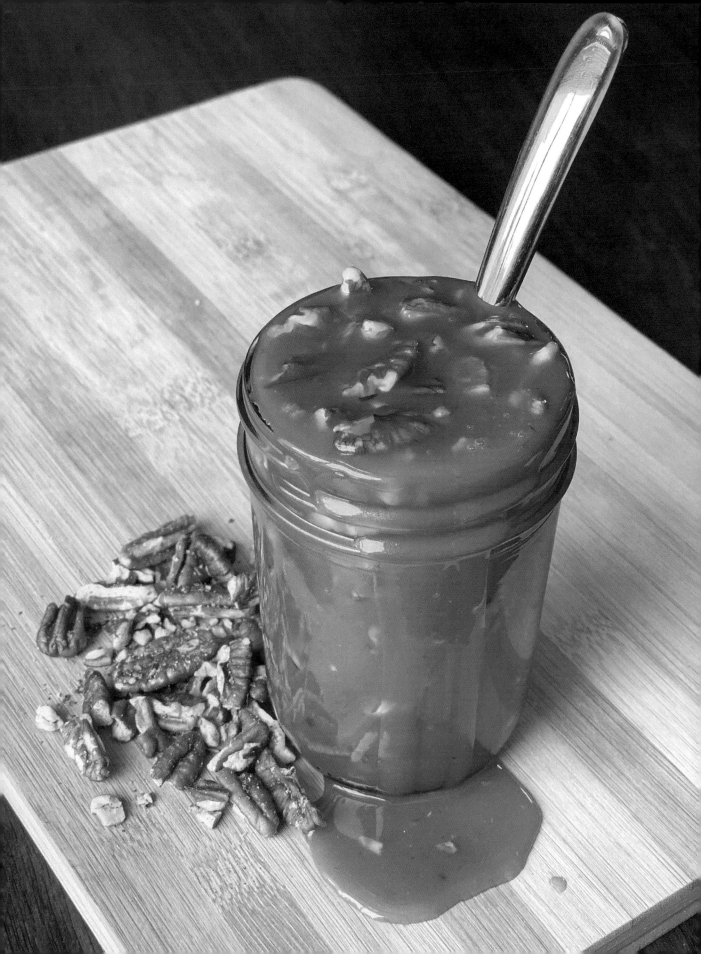

Prep Time: 3 minutes
Cook Time: 8 minutes
Yield: 16 servings
(2 tablespoons each)

BUTTERY BOURBON SAUCE

Ingredients

8 tablespoons butter
¾ cup Swerve brown sugar replacement
½ teaspoon vanilla extract
¼ cup heavy whipping cream
2 tablespoons bourbon

Directions

1. In a small saucepan, melt butter on low heat. Mix in brown sugar replacement and cook for 5 minutes while stirring.
2. Add the vanilla, heavy whipping cream, and bourbon and cook for an additional 3-4 minutes while stirring.
3. Once the caramel has thickened, remove from heat and serve on top of keto ice cream, keto pancakes/waffles, or your favorite mug cake.
4. Store in airtight container in the refrigerator for up to 2 weeks.

LET'S GET SAUCY

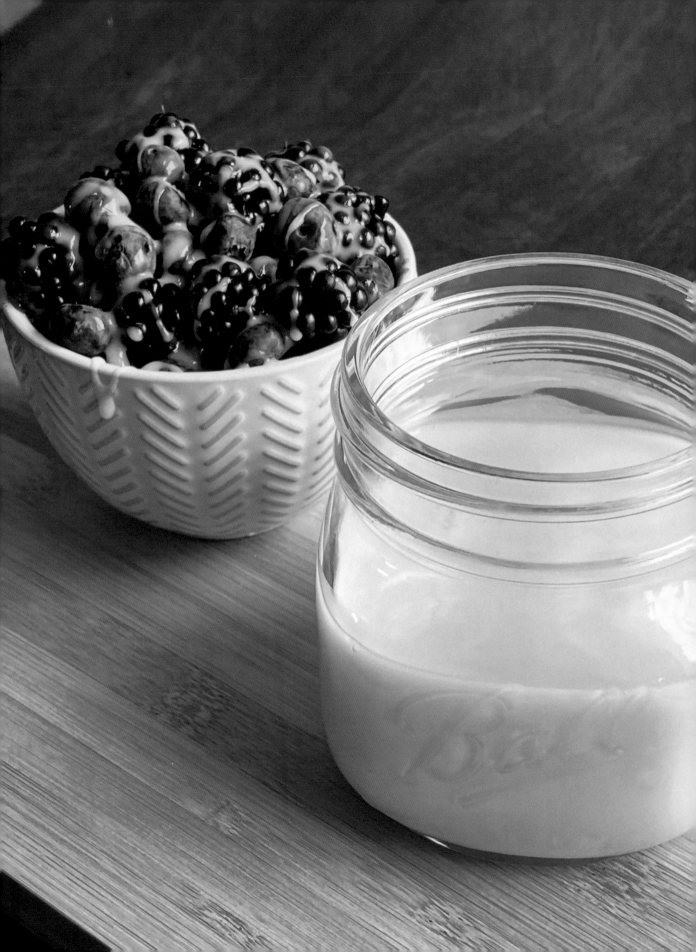

Prep Time: 30 minutes
Cook Time: 10 minutes
Yield: 12 servings
(¼ cup)

SWEETENED CONDENSED MILK

Ingredients

4 tablespoons butter
2 ½ cups heavy whipping cream
½ cup powdered sweetener
1 teaspoon vanilla extract

Directions

1. In a medium saucepan, whisk together butter and cream and bring to a simmer on medium-low heat.
2. Stir in the powdered sweetener.
3. Allow mixture to simmer for 30 minutes. The mixture will start to thicken after about 15 minutes.
4. At the 30-minute mark remove from heat and add vanilla. Whisk to combine and allow mixture to cool before storing in an airtight container.
5. Store in the refrigerator for up to a week.

EVERY LA

Tipsy Arnold Palmer

Cosmo

Margarita

Lemon Blueberry

Mojito

ST DROP

Spiked Mexican Hot Chocolate

Caribbean Rum Punch

Dirty Girl Martini

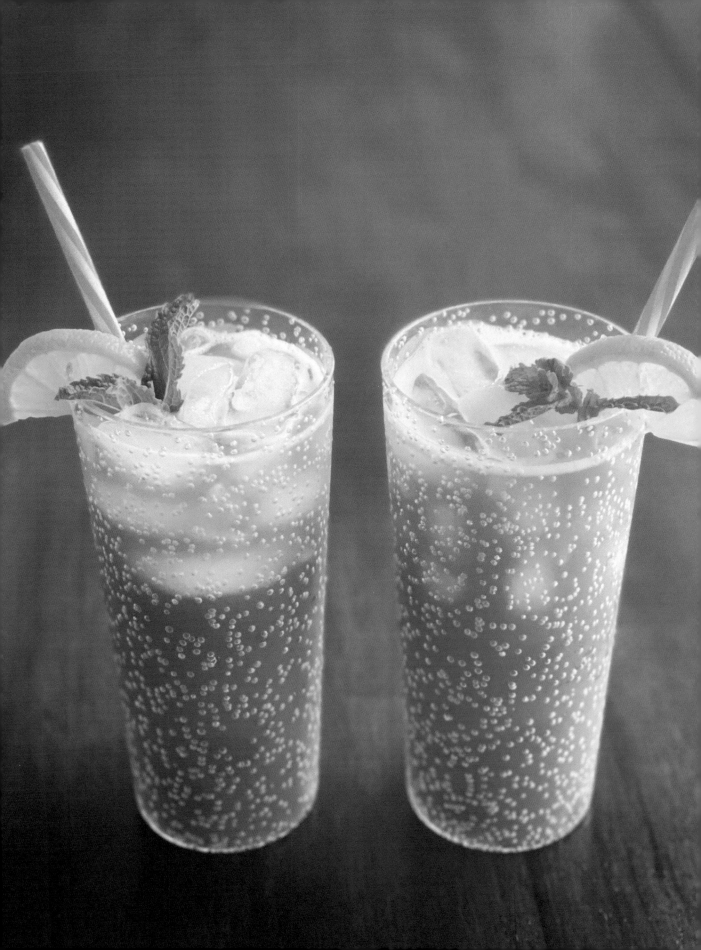

Prep Time: 3 minutes
Cook Time: 0 minutes
Yield: 1 serving

TIPSY ARNOLD PALMER

Ingredients

4 ounces unsweetened black tea, chilled
3 ounces vodka
2 ounces lemon juice
Ice
2 squeezes liquid monk fruit sweetener or stevia
Lemon wheel and mint for garnish

Directions

1. Fill a shaker cup halfway with ice. Add cold tea, vodka, lemon juice, and liquid sweetener. Shake well.
2. Pour in a tall glass over ice.
3. Garnish with fresh lemon wheel and mint.

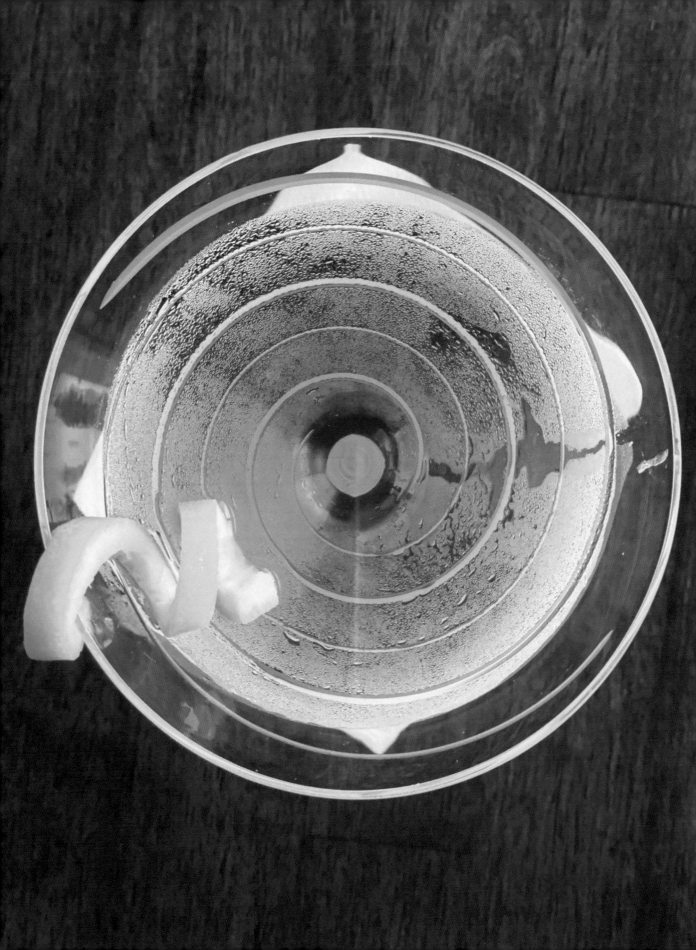

COSMO

Ingredients

Ice
3 ounces vodka
2 squeezes of liquid monk fruit sweetener or stevia
½ ounce triple sec
1 ounce no-sugar-added cranberry juice
½ ounce fresh lime juice
1 teaspoon no-sugar-added orange juice
Lime wheel for garnish

Directions

1. Add all the ingredients, except the lime wheel, to a shaker cup filled with ice and shake well.
2. Strain into a martini glass.
3. Add lime wheel to the rim of the glass and enjoy.

EVERY LAST DROP

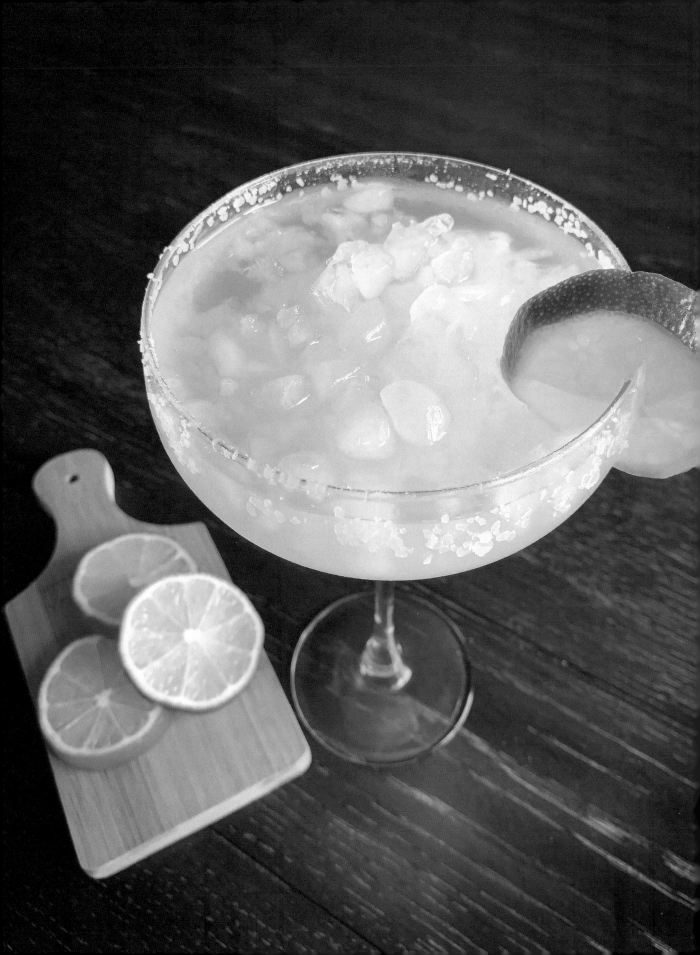

Prep Time: 3 minutes
Cook Time: 0 minutes
Yield: 1 serving

MARGARITA

Ingredients

Ice

3 ounces tequila

2 ounces fresh lime juice

2 squeezes of liquid monk fruit sweetener or stevia

Lime wheel and salt for garnish

Directions

1. Add all the ingredients to a shaker cup and shake well.
2. Strain into a margarita glass filled with ice.
3. Garnish the rim of the glass with salt and a lime wheel.

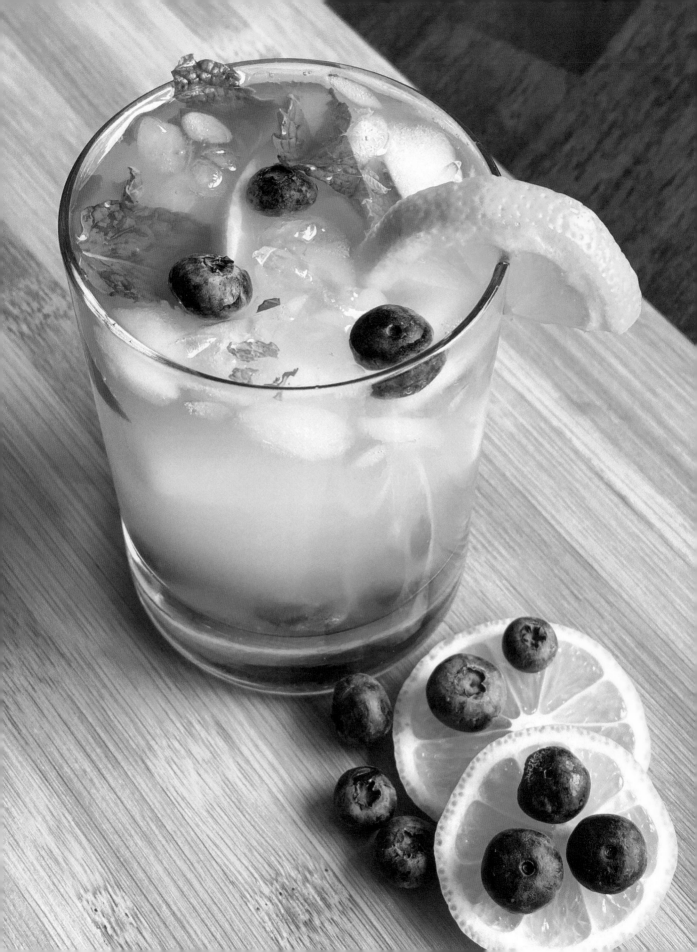

Prep Time: 5 minutes
Cook Time: 0 minutes
Yield: 1 serving

LEMON BLUEBERRY MOJITO

Ingredients

3-5 fresh mint leaves
4 blueberries
Ice
2-3 tablespoons lemon juice
2-3 squirts sugar-free sweetener
3 ounces white rum
½ cup club soda

Directions

1. Muddle mint leaves and blueberries in a shaker cup.
2. Add ice, lemon juice, sweetener, and rum. Shake well.
3. Pour into a glass filled with ice and top with club soda and garnish with a fresh mint leaf.

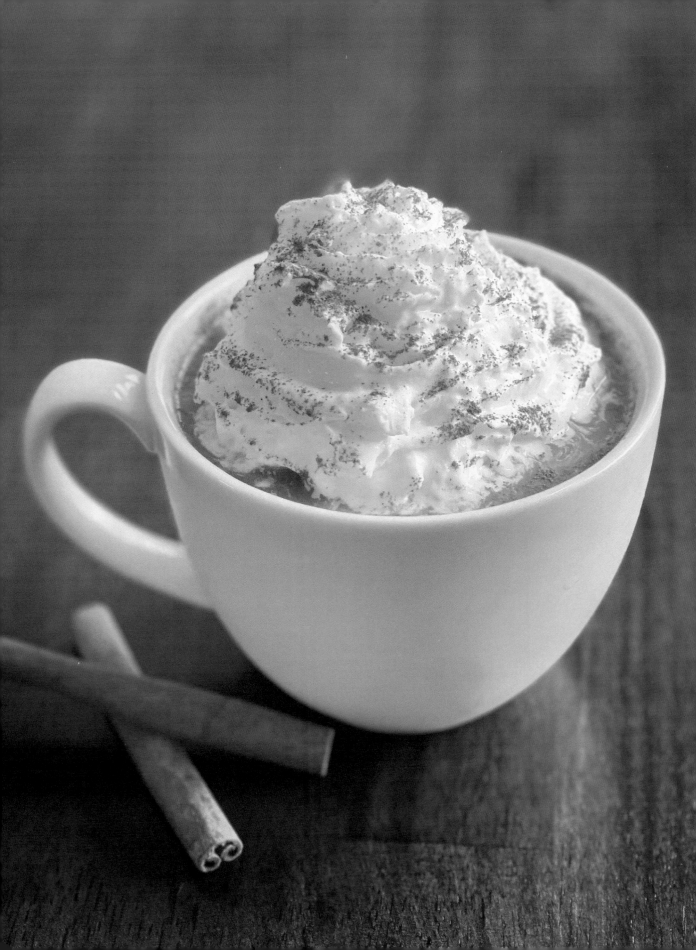

Prep Time: 3 minutes
Cook Time: 5 minutes
Yield: 1 serving

SPIKED MEXICAN HOT CHOCOLATE

Ingredients

½ cup heavy whipping cream
½ cup half & half
2 tablespoons unsweetened cocoa powder
½ teaspoon ground cinnamon
⅛ teaspoon vanilla extract
6-10 drops of liquid monk fruit or stevia
1 ½ ounces spiced rum
Whipped cream for topping

Directions

1. In a medium saucepan, whisk together the heavy whipping cream, half & half, cocoa powder, cinnamon, vanilla extract, and liquid sweetener. Bring to a low simmer.
2. Add spiced rum and remove from heat.
3. Pour into a mug, top with whipped cream and a dash of cinnamon.

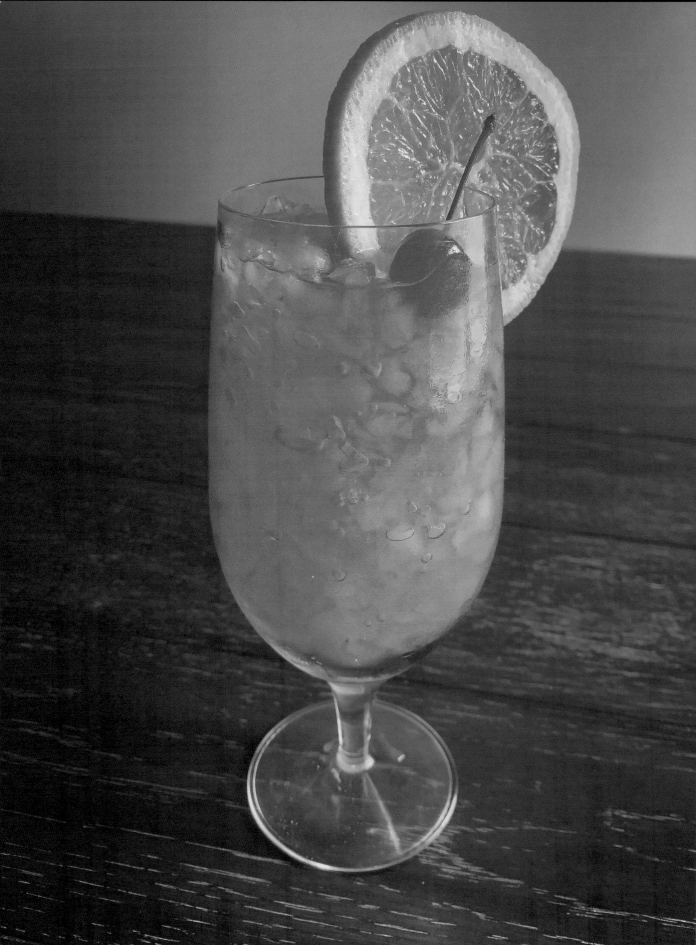

Prep Time: 3 minutes
Cook Time: 0 minutes
Yield: 1 serving

CARIBBEAN RUM PUNCH

Ingredients

3 ounces white rum
1 12-ounce can of diet Fresca or 7-Up
1 squeeze fruit punch water enhancer
Ice

Directions

1. Fill a tall glass with ice.
2. Pour in rum, soda, and fruit punch water enhancer.
3. Stir to combine and enjoy.

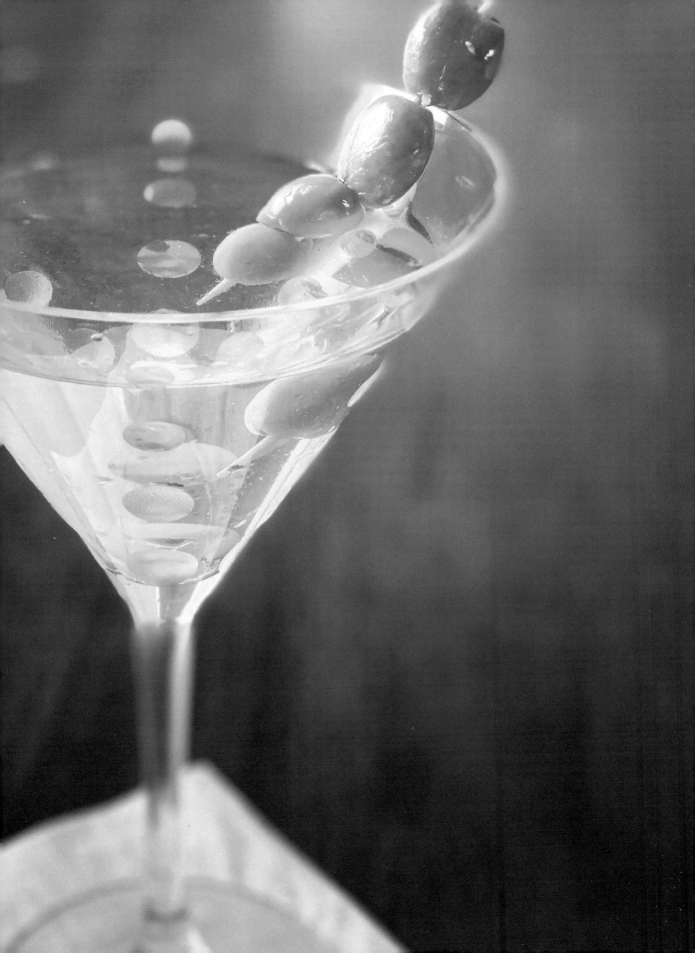

Prep Time: 3 minutes
Cook Time: 0 minutes
Yield: 1 serving

DIRTY GIRL MARTINI

Ingredients

Ice
3 ounces vodka, chilled
1 ½ ounces dry vermouth
½ ounce green olive juice
3 garlic-stuffed olives for garnish

Directions

1. Add ice to a shaker cup and pour in vodka, dry vermouth, and olive juice.
2. Shake well.
3. Strain into a martini glass and garnish with 3 olives, speared with a toothpick.

RECIPE

INDEX

WALK OF SHAME

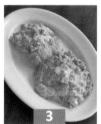
Biscuits & Gravy

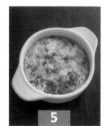
Pizza Baked Eggs

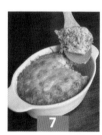
Breakfast Casserole

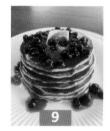
Pancake Stack with Blueberry Compote

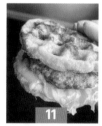
Waffle-wich

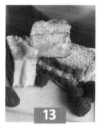
Stuffed French Toast

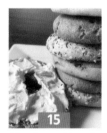
Blueberry Bagels Everything Bagels Gingerbread Bagels

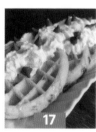
Banana Chocolate Chip Waffles

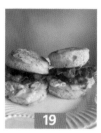
Bacon, Egg, and Cheese McMorning After

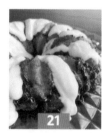
Monkey Bread

LANCE

TEASE ME

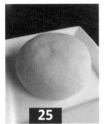
25 Fathead Dough

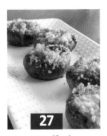
27 Stuffed Mushrooms

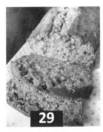
29 Zucchini Bread

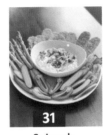
31 Spinach, Artichoke, and Jalapeño Dip

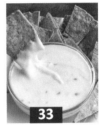
33 Queso Blanco

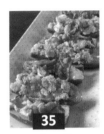
35 Jalapeño Poppers

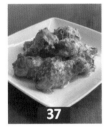
37 Maple Mustard Wings

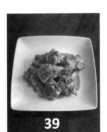
39 Sticky Peanut Butter & Jelly Wings

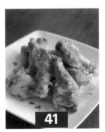
41 Garlicy Lemon Pepper Wings

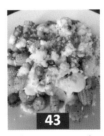
43 Elote in a Bowl

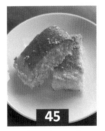
45 Cornbread

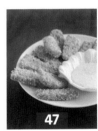
47 Ride 'Em Cowboy Pickles

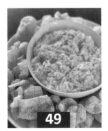
49 Jalapeño Pimento Cheese

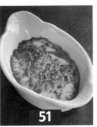
51 Oven-Baked Cheese

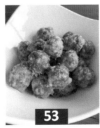
53 Party Meatballs

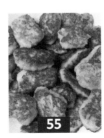
55 Faux-tato Tots

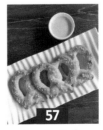
57 Jumbo Soft Pretzels

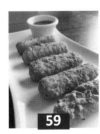
59 Fried Mozzarella Sticks

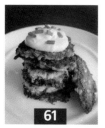
61
Zucchini Fritters

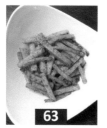
63
Jicama Fries

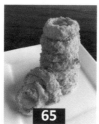
65
Onion Rings

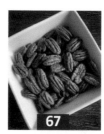
67
Party Pecans

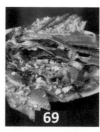
69
Chocolate Dipped Bacon
Pecan Praline Bacon
Bourbon Candied Bacon

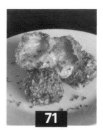
71
Fried Pimento Cheese Balls

EAT ME

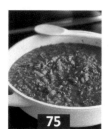
75
Chili

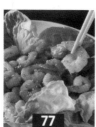
77
Bang Bang (Between the Sheets) Shrimp

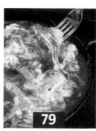
79
Meatball Bake

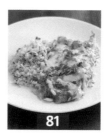
81
White Chicken Enchiladas

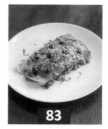
83
Red Rendezvous Pork Enchiladas

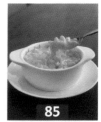
85
Creamy Macaroni & Cheese

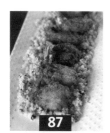
87
Coconut Shrimp with Cilantro-Lime Cauli-Rice

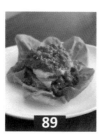
89
Chili Cheeseburger

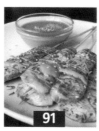
91
Chicken Satay with Peanut Sauce

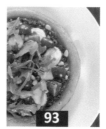
93
Pesto Pizza

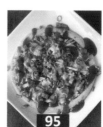
95
BBQ Chicken Pizza

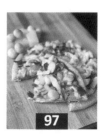
97
Nutty Hawaiian Pizza

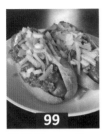

99

Chili Cheese Dog

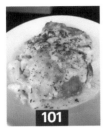

101

Zucchini Au Gratin

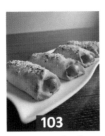

103

Pigs in a Blanket

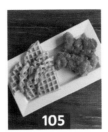

105

Chicken 'n Waffles

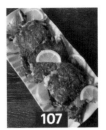

107

Crab Cakes

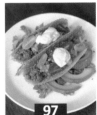

97

Crispy Cheese Shell Tacos

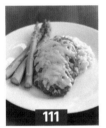

111

Chicken Parmesan

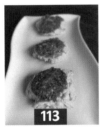

113

Buffalo Chicken Patties

WHIPPED & CREAMED

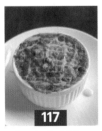

117

Apple Cobbler

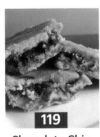

119

Chocolate Chip Pecan Pie Bars

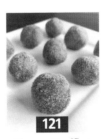

121

Churro Truffles

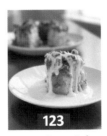

123

Butter Rum Cake

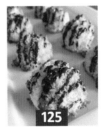

125

Coconut Macaroons

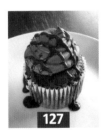

127

Chocolate Cupcakes with Chocolate Buttercream

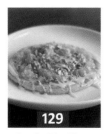
Apple Pie Pizza

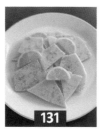
Crema de Limón Bark

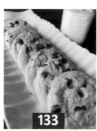
Chocolate Chip Cookies

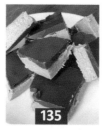
No-Bake Quickie Peanut Butter Bars

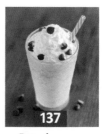
Grasshopper Milkshake

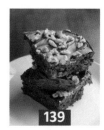
Fudgy as F*ck Ganache Brownies

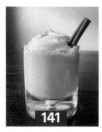
Pumpkin Mousse with Spiced Whipped Cream

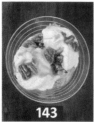
Vanilla Bean Ice Cream with Buttery Bourbon Sauce

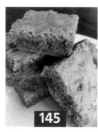
Peanut Butter Blondies

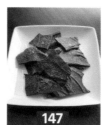
Sweet & Spicy Midnight Bark

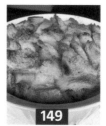
Vanilla Rum Bread Pudding

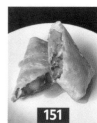
Apple Turn-(Me)-Over

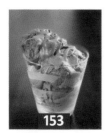
Chocolate Peanut Butter Ice Cream

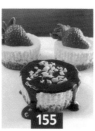
Cheesecake Bites

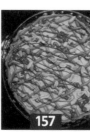
Peanut Butter Pie

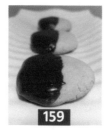
Tuxedo Shortbread Cookies

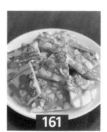
White Chocolate Peanut Butter Bark

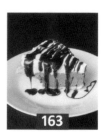
French Silk Pie

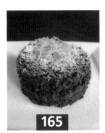

Chocolate Orange Mug Cake 165

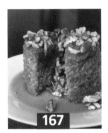

Maple Pecan Spice Mug Cake 167

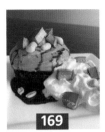

Chocolate Peanut Butter Mug Cake 169

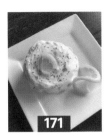

Lemon Poppy Seed Mug Cake 171

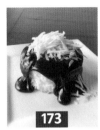

Cocoa Bunny Mug Cake 173

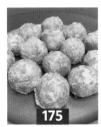

Russian Tea Cakes 175

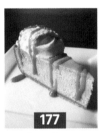

Drunken Pumpkin Cheesecake 177

LET'S GET SAUCY

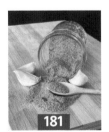

Taco Seasoning 181

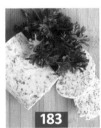

Basil, Parmesan, Parsley Butter 183

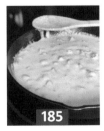

Country Gravy 185

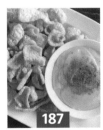

Beer Cheese 187

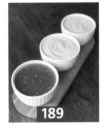

Sriracha Sauce Bang Bang Sauce Shishido Pepper Sauce 189

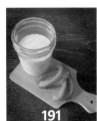

Everyday Ranch 191

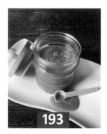

193

Salted Caramel
Sauce

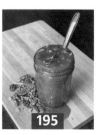

195

Buttery Bourbon
Sauce

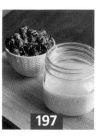

197

Sweetened
Condensed Milk

EVERY LAST DROP

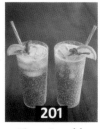

201

Tipsy Arnold
Palmer

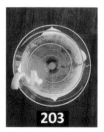

203

Cosmo

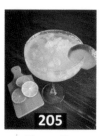

205

Margarita

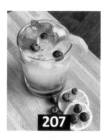

207

Lemon Blueberry
Mojito

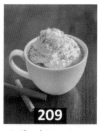

209

Spiked Mexican
Hot Chocolate

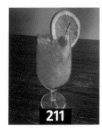

211

Caribbean Rum
Punch

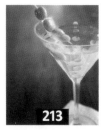

213

Dirty Girl Martini

Follow Erika Rivera on Instagram for more recipes.
www.instagram.com/lowcarbwitherika

Follow E.K. Blair on Instagram for more recipes.
www.instagram.com/ek.blair

Check out E.K. Blair's fiction books.
www.ekblair.com/books

CPSIA information can be obtained at www.ICGtesting.com
Printed in the USA
LVIW012329121120
671603LV00011B/116